"The most significant part of the book is the step-by-step instructions you can follow at home in order to teach yourself to have orgasms . . . A woman can learn in an amazingly short time how to have orgasms. The women seen in our clinical practice, on which this book is based, have proved this to be true in spite of years of negative sexual conditioning . . . We would like to see an end to the misery of every one of those women who are not able to achieve orgasm, so that nobody need suffer from this widespread problem."

—*Georgia Kline-Graber*
Benjamin Graber

D0834195

About the Authors

BENJAMIN GRABER, M.D., and GEORGIA KLINE-GRABER, R.N., live with their son in Madison, Wisconsin, where they operate a medical clinic for the treatment of sexual dysfunction. Prior to that they were in private practice for three years at the Sexual Therapy Medical Clinic in Marina del Rey, California. Together they have written numerous articles for general magazines and professional journals, and appeared on many radio and television shows, including their own weekly National Public Radio program, "Sexual Re-education."

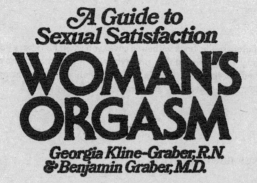

A Guide to
Sexual Satisfaction

WOMAN'S ORGASM

Georgia Kline-Graber, R.N.
& Benjamin Graber, M.D.

WARNER BOOKS

A Time Warner Company

WARNER BOOKS EDITION

This Warner Books Edition is published by arrangement with Bobbs-Merrill Company, Inc.
Box 558
4300 West 62nd Street
Indianapolis, Indiana 46206

Warner Books, Inc.
1271 Avenue of the Americas
New York, N.Y. 10020

A Time Warner Company

Printed in the United States of America

First Warner Books Printing: June, 1983

15   14   13   12

To our patients—past, present and future

ACKNOWLEDGMENTS

No contribution to the field of human sexuality arises out of a vacuum. We owe a debt to those courageous pioneers Sigmund Freud, Havelock Ellis, T. H. Van de Velde, R. L. Dickinson, Alfred Kinsey, and others not so renowned, who opened the early pathways of communication. Modern researchers such as William Masters, M.D.; Virginia Johnson; Helen Kaplan, M.D., Ph.D.; and Mary Jane Sherfey, M.D., have continued to enlarge upon the knowledge so necessary for the understanding of the human sexual condition.

Two individuals are especially important to the development of this work. The late Arnold Kegel, M.D., Associate Clinical Professor of Gynecology and Obstetrics at the University of Southern California School of Medicine, was a gynecologist whose focus was a condition called stress incontinence. However, his work on the pubococcygeus muscle, although currently known and recognized primarily by gynecologists and professionals in the field of sexuality, has resulted in one of the most important findings of modern sexual research. We are greatly indebted to him. Our respect and appreciation also go to Joseph LoPiccolo, Ph.D., currently at State University of New York, Stony Brook, who developed the step-by-step program for the treatment of female orgasmic dysfunction on which this book as well as other programs in the country, is based.

Joseph Oliver, M.D.; Arthur Schapiro, M.D.; Anthony T. Schnurer, M.D.; James Semmens, M.D.; Jane Semmens; Howard Shapiro, M.D.; and Leonard Zunin, M.D., all aided in the development of our professional skills, and their help and support of our work at the clinic are deeply appreciated. Grateful appreciation also goes to Mary McKendry, R.N., Instructor of Nursing at Santa Monica College, who taught her students to assume nothing, to question everything, and then to question it again. Our deepest personal thanks goes to Lawrence Newman, M.D., without whose encouragement, advice, and emotional support this book would not have been possible.

Our friend and former secretary, Lilian Warshawer, has consistently been one of the most wholehearted and loyal supporters of our work and has repeatedly worked early and late in order to help us out. Her unfailing dedication has been invaluable, both for the patients and for us. Diane Giddis, our editor at Bobbs-Merrill, did a meticulous and brilliant job of editing the manuscript, understanding what women might need from the book and giving it her consistent and enthusiastic support. We also wish to thank our much loved son Michael, age ten, who did without his parents on many occasions while we were working on the research and writing the manuscript.

We are grateful to Dr. Kegel's daughter-in-law, Millie Kegel, and to his former secretary, Jane Fones, who provided help and information concerning his work. We wish to thank Lou Riggs of KCRW-FM radio and Mark Bragg of Public Affairs Broadcast Group for their encouragement and belief in our work and for helping us to present sex education to the public in a serious and professional manner. We also wish to thank the following friends who have helped us in various ways: Mark Edelstein, Susan Edelstein, Fran Howard, Lloyd Kaechle, Lou Marston, Michael Walley, and Dave Zaslow. James Ludlum, Harriet Pilpel, and Laurie Rockett all provided excellent legal advice in a warm and human manner. And our parents, Dodie Ramsey, Robert Kline, Cecil Graber and Louis Graber, as well as Mary Kline, have given us their consistent admiration and encouragement.

Lastly, of course, we are forever indebted to the more than one thousand patients who over the last three years have allowed us the privilege of sharing in their lives, their problems, their pain and their joys. The memory of them will be with us always.

TABLE OF CONTENTS

PART 4 *The Road to the Future*

WOMAN'S ORGASM

Preface

This book is not a novel, but it has thousands of heroines. It is dedicated to those courageous women across the country who have passed through the doors of our clinic and others, looking for answers. Some are angry and frustrated at continually having to answer "No" to the inevitable question, "Did you come?" Others suffer a private shame for years of deceit at faking their climax. Their question is always the same: "Why can't I have an orgasm?"

As medical therapists we are greatly concerned about this problem. It has become clear to us that nobody knows for sure how many women actually suffer from this lack of sexual satisfaction. At our former private practice, the Sexual Therapy Medical Clinic in Los Angeles, we interviewed over one thousand patients who came to the clinic with various sexual problems. Some of the women seen came in knowing they had difficulty with orgasm, whereas others either came in with other sexual problems or were accompanying their husbands or male partners who had the sexual difficulty. By questioning these women in our clinical practice, we learned to our dismay that many women do not even know what an orgasm feels like. This fact throws into serious question all available statistics on the number of women suffering from this problem. Every day at the clinic a woman who thought she was having orgasms would tell us, after intensive questioning by a female therapist who is herself able to have an orgasm, "If that's what an orgasm feels like, then I guess I've never really had one." Many women think they are having orgasms but aren't really sure. Others who think they are not having orgasms actually are.

Whatever the actual incidence of orgasmic dysfunction, it is undoubtedly high. However, we have found in our practice that it is lack of knowledge, not psychiatric problems, that prevents most women from having orgasms. Just as most women are not taught either directly or indirectly how to throw a football, neither are they "taught" how to have an orgasm. Orgasm stripped of romance (which we do only to simplify this explanation) is a physiological event that involves nerves and muscles and the coordination of the two. Just as an adult woman could learn how to throw a football with some skill if she wanted to, so can she also learn in an amazingly short time how to have orgasms. The women seen in our clinical practice, on which this book is based, have proved this to be true in spite of the years of negative sexual conditioning they have endured.

In addition to providing a definition of what an orgasm is and what it feels like, we discuss in this book previously published information relating to female sexuality, physiological facts about male and female sexual response, and the actual specific medical problems that interfere with a woman's ability to achieve orgasm and how they can be corrected by her doctor. But the most significant part of the book is the step-by-step instructions you can follow at home in order to teach yourself how to have orgasms, both alone and with intercourse.

Learning is growth, and growth is change. Our hope is that this book will in some way change your life by teaching you to have orgasms. It is always frustrating to a therapist to realize that for each person who is helped in the clinic, there are hundreds of others who need and desperately want help but cannot afford the time or money necessary to obtain treatment. Daily we are given reminders of the unhappiness caused by sexual dissatisfaction. We would like to see an end to the misery of every one of those unfortunate women who are not able to achieve orgasm, so that nobody need suffer from this widespread and devastating problem.

We are dedicated to continuing the medical clinical investigation and practice of sexual diagnosis and treatment. *Woman's Orgasm* is a report on one small aspect of that goal. We hope that it will help.

G.K-G.
B.G.
Madison, Wisconsin

PART 1

Description of
Female Orgasm

Many women continually ask themselves, "Do I or don't I have orgasms?" A cloud of mystery still surrounds the female orgasm, or climax, in spite of all that has been written on the subject. Every day at the clinic at least one woman is embarrassed to admit that she is not sure whether she is having orgasms or not. And it is probably not unfair to say that this woman represents hundreds to thousands of others who secretly have the same doubts but are afraid to voice them.

Sadly, most women do not dare to ask even close friends or relatives about their sexual experiences. They consider such a step impolite at best and in any case fraught with embarrassment. The woman who does ask often receives answers that confirm her fear that she is the only woman in the world having trouble, and she is left with instructions to "just relax and do what comes naturally." No description of orgasm is offered—only reassurances that she'll "know when it happens." She never finds out, and it never happens.

Turning to professional help is also often unrewarding

for women. Most physicians and therapists in this country are men, so none of them have ever experienced a female orgasm. And of those therapists who are female, unfortunately many are non-orgasmic themselves. Although a female therapist may be more empathic, she will be of limited helpfulness unless she herself is orgasmic.

Widespread lack of information on exactly what an orgasm feels like causes confusion and makes it even harder to achieve.

A major factor that has prevented women from understanding their own orgasm has been the uncertainty over where the orgasm takes place. This is largely a result of the controversy between the so-called clitoral and the so-called vaginal orgasm.

In order to understand orgasm, consider what happens when your doctor taps your knee with a little rubber hammer. What takes place is known as a reflex. This reflex has two basic parts: the incoming sensation, known as the *sensory input,* which is the tap of the hammer; and the result, described as the *motor or muscular output,* when the leg jumps.

With female orgasm, theoretically the incoming sensation can result from being touched anywhere on the body—for example the breast—but usually involves primarily the clitoris, the little pea-sized structure that is found at the upper junction of the inner lips of the vagina (Figure 1, facing page 39) and in the woman is the counterpart of the head of the penis in the man. With intercourse, it is the pubococcygeus muscle in the vagina that is receiving direct stimulation, while the clitoris usually receives only indirect stimulation.

The pubococcygeus muscle, a strong band of muscle about three-fourths to one inch wide when fully developed and healthy, is located three to five centimeters beyond the entrance of the unstimulated vagina and runs around it, in the manner of something encircling a tube. It is attached to the pubic bone in the front and the coccyx (tailbone) in the back. It runs like a thick rubber band from the pubic bone to either side of the urethra and part of the bladder, to either side of the middle of the vagina, and to either side of the large intestine, to the coccyx. Each time you hold back on urinating, it is the pubococcygeus muscle you are contracting. And each time you squeeze your vagina together, you contract the same pubococcygeus muscle. The healthy muscle is firm to the touch, and strong.

When enough sensation has been experienced or has built up from whatever source, orgasm occurs. Pursuing the knee-tapping example, the "jerk" occurs when the tap of the hammer is in the right place and is forceful enough. Too light a tap and the leg does not jump. Although the incoming sensation may come from a variety of sources, the orgasm itself always occurs *inside the body,* in the vagina, or, more precisely, in the pubococcygeus muscle. The contractions of this muscle correspond to the leg's jumping, and are identical to the ones that occur in male orgasm which result in ejaculation, the spurting of fluid containing sperm. These muscular contractions are the hallmark of orgasm—male or female—and occur regardless of how the orgasm is initiated: whether from primarily clitorial stimulation, from a combination of clitoral and pubococcygeal stimulation, or from primarily pubococcygeal stimulation. They are often quite distinct, and without them *there has been no orgasm.*

There are, however, differences in the way the orgasm and vaginal contractions feel *physically,* depending on whether or not there is something inserted in the vagina during orgasm (such as an orgasm with intercourse). Obviously there are emotional differences as well between, for example, an orgasm experienced in intercourse and a clitorally induced orgasm experienced in masturbation, but the physical sensations need to be understood first. Although some women masturbate with something inserted in the vagina, it is easier first to describe how an orgasm feels with only direct clitoral stimulation, such as during masturbation.

When a women receives only direct clitoral stimulation, she experiences very pleasant tingling sensations that slowly build up to orgasm. As she nears orgasm, the tingling sensations become more and more intense. As orgasm becomes imminent, her attention is focused on what is happening with her body. All other sensations—sounds, tastes, smells, etc.—are diminished.

The first distinct stage or step of the actual orgasm is a feeling of stoppage or suspension. It lasts only an instant and is quickly followed by the second stage: the sensations in the clitoris disappear and are superseded by a feeling of warmth and tingling throughout the entire pelvis (even though it is the clitoris that is receiving direct stimulation) and sometimes, with a really intense orgasm, in other parts of the body as well. The pelvis becomes flooded with a warm, heavy, sexual sensation which then becomes the most distinct feeling, taking over from the sensations in the clitoris alone. In reality this feeling lasts for only about five seconds, but it seems much longer. Often there is a feeling of almost floating, and one is unaware of touching anything, such as a blanket or a pillow. Attention is riveted on experiencing the sensation, and outside distractions are easily ignored.

The last stage occurs after a split-second pause following the feelings described above. Automatically, the pubococcygeus muscle contracts strongly, bringing the sides of the vagina together. With this contraction of the muscle, there is the same delicious feeling described above. As the muscle relaxes, the feeling stops, but the motion of the muscle relaxing or opening is felt as a movement. The time of this pause has been measured at 0.8 second. Then the muscle contracts again with the same sensations.

An average orgasm will consist of three or four contractions; an intense orgasm can contain up to about fifteen contractions. With very intense orgasms the warm, tingling feelings are apparent not only as the muscle contracts or closes but also as it opens (sometimes through two or three contractions).

If a woman experiences a continuous sensation of warmth and tingling but not the contractions, she is not having an orgasm, although she is quite close. The sensations of warmth and tingling before the contractions are a pre-orgasmic phenomenon and are equivalent to the "ejaculatory inevitability period" in a man.[1] (This is the point just before ejaculation occurs and is a sensation that most men can identify.) The automatic vaginal contractions are the actual physiological orgasm; they are not to be confused with the pulsation in the clitoral area, which is caused by increased blood in the pelvis due to excitation. Although the waves of sensation are usually recognized by the woman who is having an orgasm, it is often difficult for her to localize these feelings to the vagina, or, more specifically, to the pubococcygeus muscle. At the clinic, after the physiology of orgasm has been explained and the woman has an understanding of the pubococcygeus muscle, she can usually then localize the phenomenon of the waves of feeling to the pelvis and the vaginal muscle, where the waves are originating. It is important to re-emphasize that the orgasm described above is one initiated by clitorial stimulation alone but which physiologically occurs and can be felt in the pubococcygeus muscle.

The orgasm with intercourse is basically the same but does have a few very important differences. The reason for these differences is twofold: first, the initial or incoming stimulation occurs primarily in the pubococcygeus muscle in the vagina; and secondly, when the contractions occur, there is something in the vagina, namely the penis. When a woman is having intercourse, she experiences most of the feelings in the vaginal area instead of the clitoris, provided the man is thrusting or she is moving properly. The clitoris is in fact getting some stimulation *indirectly* in any position used, but even so she does not feel most of this clitoral stimulation. The walls of the vagina itself have very few nerve endings, but the muscle that lies underneath the wall—the pubococcygeus—is replete with nerve endings. The condition of this muscle determines how much sensation the woman experiences with vaginal stimulation. If the muscle is in good condition, it is more likely there will be a sufficient amount of sensation for orgasm to occur. Again, stimulation of the muscle acts like a tap of the hammer on the knee: if enough stimulation is received, orgasm occurs.

This orgasm also is preceded by a buildup in sensation and begins with an instant of stoppage or suspension of time. Again this is followed by the flash-flood of delicious, warm, tingling feeling. The focus of feeling switches to the entire pelvis and then sometimes to the rest of the body. This sensation, as previously described, lasts about five seconds but feels much longer. Even though the woman is making contact with her lover's body, she is largely unaware of his presence and is engulfed in her own sensations. It is almost impossible to distract her at this time. Again, as with the clitorally induced orgasm, the flood of feeling is followed by a brief pause, and then the third stage occurs—the contractions of the pubococcygeus muscle.

With intercourse, however, the contractions feel less intense and more subtle. They are experienced as flicks of movement instead of the distinct contractions described above with clitoral masturbation. Many women describe this as a fluttering sensation in the vagina. The reason for the difference is that the penis is holding the vaginal walls apart. The vaginal contractions occur against the penis, which prevents the walls from moving together with the same intensity. The actual movement of the muscle as measured in the laboratory is not as great,[2] and the sensation for the woman is consequently less distinct.

Not all nerves and nerve endings are the same. Some nerve endings are stimulated or "triggered" by hot or cold, some by the sharp point of a pin; others are triggered only by dull pressure. The nerve endings found in the vaginal muscle are a special kind, called "proprioceptive" or pressure-sensitive, found in muscles and joints. What these specialized receivers "feel" is how little or how much a muscle moves. Therefore, during intercourse, when the penis is inserted in the vagina between the two parts of the muscle, the nerve endings "feel" less movement with each contraction, and the intensity of the orgasm is decreased.

It is true that many women prefer sexual activity with a partner and find orgasm with intercourse more *emotionally* satisfying than one without, particularly within the context of a love relationship. However, the orgasm that occurs without the penis inside feels more distinct on a *physical* basis because it is physically more intense.[3]

In summary, female orgasm by any form of stimulation consists of a distinct abrupt stoppage of time, followed by a suffusion of warmth and tingling, followed by a series of automatic contractions of the pubococcygeus muscle in the vagina. There are subtle variations on the basic theme as elaborated above, but this is the essence of an orgasm.

PART 2

The Problem

CHAPTER 1

Physiology of Orgasm

One of the most common criticisms leveled at sexual therapists is that they reduce sex to mechanics, stripping it of romance. For unknown reasons, people have expectations from sex that they would consider ridiculous in any other physical human endeavor. No one would attempt to build a house without first learning the basics of carpentry. Beethoven began with the same scales that every student learns in music class. Yet people expect to be able to perform great sexual feats even though they are ignorant of the basic facts that underlie them.

In order to understand and enjoy lovemaking, it is important to learn about basic anatomy and the physiology of sex. Once the musician learns the scales, he does not think of them each time he begins to play, yet his underlying knowledge is what allows him to perform with confidence. The same is true of the lover. As long as the biology of sex is a mystery, mysterious forces can rob him of his potency or deprive her of her orgasm. Once the basics have been learned, sonatas and symphonies can be created.

Unfortunately, one of the biggest gaps in our educational system is in the area of human sexuality. If there is any sex education at all, it is usually about how sperm meets egg and not about how to make love with another human being.

The following information is a review of the sexual response cycle as elaborated by Masters and Johnson. Understanding this will help you in using the self-help portion of this book. We are also including this information in order to point out the false assumptions society has made over differences in anatomy and physiology between men and women. The roles that boys and girls, men and women, automatically assume in society have been one of the chief reasons of female sexual problems. As far as sexuality goes, male and female responses are practically identical—not, as many theories try to prove, completely different.

Modern embryology, in fact, has uncovered a startling fact which totally contradicts ancient theology and the "Eve came from Adam's rib" myth. It turns out that the basic human organism is female. If there were no hormonal intervention, every fetus that developed in the uterus would be born with female genitals and female reproductive organs. But if the chromosomes, which carry the genetic message, dictate that the fetus is to be a boy, then testosterone, a hormone, must be secreted in order for the basic female embryo to be converted into a male.[1]

Some feminists have used this information to demonstrate the natural superiority of women. Instead of using it to compete, one can more usefully see this common beginning as suggestive of the similarity of men and women.

In normal male genital anatomy, the penis consists of three erectile bodies: two corpus cavernosa and the corpus spongiosum. The testicles are contained in the scrotum, which actually is formed during the development of the fetus in the uterus by the fusion of the two labia majora.

A reminder of the common origin of male and female anatomy can be seen by tracing the path of the spermatic tubules, which begin at the testes but return into the abdomen and eventually find their way into the prostate. The path of these tubes illustrates the fact that the precursors of the testes resided in the abdomen, as do the ovaries in the female. The spermatic tubules empty into the prostate, and the sperm pass through the ejaculatory ducts into the urethra and subsequently through the end of the penis.

In normal female anatomy, the homologue of the penis, the clitoris, is much smaller in size but also consists of erectile tissue. It has a head or glans and a shaft, just like its homologue. The clitoris, like the uncircumcised penis, also has a foreskin or prepuce. Although the clitoris is smaller on the surface than the penis, its vascular extensions are pervasive in the labial folds and underneath.

In elaborating the sexual response cycle, Masters and Johnson arbitrarily divided it into four phases: excitement, plateau, orgasm, and resolution.[2] Essentially, two bodily reactions are consistent throughout the entire sexual process. As excitement builds, the sexual organs become engorged with blood (vaso-congestion), and the accessory muscles tighten. The best non-genital example is a sneeze. Remember what it feels like to sneeze and you will have a basic understanding of the physiology of an orgasm. With a sneeze the face fills up with blood, so that it is temporarily suffused with warmth. Then the muscles tighten, and suddenly the sneeze occurs with explosive force, the extra blood rushes out of the face and the muscles relax.

The most obvious genital example of this process is the erection of the penis. As the penis fills with blood, it erects, and its suspensory muscles tighten and cause it to rise from its overhanging position. A lesser-known fact is that the clitoris also erects during sexual excitement, and a tremendous amount of blood rushes to the female pelvis, as it does to the male penis. As explained above, the homologous vasculature in the female lies in and under the labia and outer one-third of the vagina. This increased vascular load seeps through the walls of the vagina in the form of a fluid and provides for vaginal lubrication. Besides the suffusion of blood to the clitoris, then, the female "erection" is evidenced by the appearance of the vaginal lubrication, which occurs within seconds after the woman becomes aroused.[8]

Other changes occur at this point. In the man the testicles begin to elevate toward the body, and in the female the labia enlarge as a result of the increased blood flow mentioned above and begin to form a tunnel-like extension to the vagina that acts as a receptacle for the penis. The vagina itself begins to lengthen and expand in size.

During the plateau stage the penis becomes fully erect and the testicles complete their elevation toward the body, while the scrotum also completes its ascent. The urethra has extended in size, as have the testicles, again due to the marked increase in blood flow into the area. During the plateau phase, the time length of which is totally variable, the penis emits some pre-coital lubrication which originates in the Cowper's gland, one of the accessory male sexual organs. This lubrication contains millions of sperm, and, since it is present well before ejaculation, it accounts for the many failures of the withdrawal method of contraception.

In the female the clitoris actually withdraws beneath its hood and becomes fairly inaccessible to direct contact. The labia minora continue to increase in size and actually undergo a color change reminiscent of the color change that some primates undergo in what has been labeled their "sex skin." The labia majora also increase in size, again due to the vasocongestion of the tissues.

The vagina has completed its expansion and is now quite different from its original size. The outer portion forms what is known as the orgasmic platform which overlies the pubococcygeus muscle, the vaginal muscle that surrounds the inlet to the vagina like a doughnut.

As described earlier, prior to orgasm there is a preliminary stage which in the male is known as the ejaculatory inevitability stage. Physiologically, during this stage the secondary sexual organs, the prostate and seminal vesicles, are contracting. In the next stage the penile muscles contract and expel the sperm. The male ejaculate that occurs with orgasm is about a teaspoon in amount and contains approximately 50 to 200 million sperm. With female orgasm the uterus contracts, but, especially important, the circumvaginal muscle contracts rhythmically and automatically, just as do the penile muscles that cause the ejaculation.

This again is a dramatic example of the similarity between male and female sexual response. Both the muscles causing male ejaculation and the circumvaginal muscle with the orgasmic platform contract at 0.8 second; both contract to the same tenth of a second! These contractions are the actual physiological sign of orgasm.

As mentioned earlier, orgasm is a sensory-motor reflex loop. Stimulation is received in the penis, breast, clitoris or elsewhere, and when enough stimulation has accumulated, orgasm occurs as a muscular response, just like the response of the leg to the tap of the doctor's reflex hammer on the knee. Without these contractions there has been no orgasm.

The muscular contractions help to expel the extra blood from the pelvis. For the woman, failure to have these would be equivalent to the male's failure to ejaculate during intercourse. The consequences are tension, discomfort, irritability, and sometimes physical symptoms such as cramps or backache. This condition is known medically as Taylor's syndrome or pelvic congestion syndrome. The greater the level of arousal, the greater discomfort a woman will usually feel if she does not experience orgasm. In general, high levels of arousal are related to longer spans of foreplay and more active and intense coital experiences.

In addition, the unfortunate woman often has other misery to bear. Remember that the prelude to orgasm is the accumulation of tremendous amounts of blood in the walls of the vagina, thus producing the vaginal lubrication. Without orgasm the blood remains and the lubrication continues. This can promote irritation, chafing, and even chronic vaginal and urinary infection. It is important to state that not all vaginal and urinary infections are caused this way, nor will these problems develop every time a woman fails to climax. However, repeated cycles of excitement that do not culminate in orgasm can cause actual physical illness.

Another parallel between male and female orgasm is that in both sexes the rectal sphincter contracts with orgasm. This is noteworthy because it firmly establishes the anus as an erogenous zone, as part of normal sexual physiology, in spite of countless religious, moral and legal prohibitions to the contrary.

The final stage of the sexual response cycle is resolution. In this stage everything returns to its normal state. The current level of knowledge shows us that the male returns to original pre-excitation levels and must begin the whole cycle anew, whereas the female may return to a plateau level and quickly have subsequent orgasms, up to fifty or more in one hour with the aid of a vibrator.

This is one area of sexual functioning where men and women do seem to vary. However, there is as yet no precise physiological or anatomical basis for this difference. In fact Kinsey's statistics reveal that ten percent of the male population are multi-orgasmic at some point in their lives, so further research may elaborate on this point and determine if this current "fact" has a true physiological explanation.

In summary, then, in the sexual response cycle the male and the female, having come from a common embryonic source, go through very similar changes which basically can be reduced to a process of vasocongestion (filling up with blood) and muscular contraction, followed by an explosive set of automatic muscular contractions and a subsequent release and relaxation.

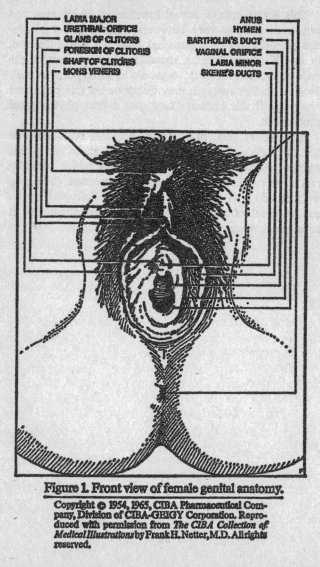

LABIA MAJOR
URETHRAL ORIFICE
GLANS OF CLITORIS
FORESKIN OF CLITORIS
SHAFT OF CLITORIS
MONS VENERIS

ANUS
HYMEN
BARTHOLIN'S DUCT
VAGINAL ORIFICE
LABIA MINOR
SKENE'S DUCTS

Figure 1. Front view of female genital anatomy.

CHAPTER 2

The Road from the Past

It is a cornerstone of wisdom that those who do not learn from the mistakes of the past are doomed to repeat them. Men and women alike must understand what has been said and thought about female sexuality and female orgasm in the past in order to understand the situation of most women today.

The past does not lack for quantity of opinion about female orgasm. Daniel G. Brown, in an excellent review of the literature on the subject, "Female Orgasm and Sexual Inadequacy," cites 167 references.[1] Seymour Fisher's book, *The Female Orgasm*, has an extensive review of commentaries on women and their sexual response and contains over 3,000 references. Yet in spite of this quantity of literature, many mysteries remain, many fallacies abound, and some of the real truths about female orgasm are yet to be clearly enunciated. As Fisher, at the conclusion of his exhaustive review of past opinions, puts it: "There seems to be good reason for questioning practically every accepted idea about femininity and placing a serious burden of proof upon anyone who declares that a woman's sexual behavior is determined by one variable rather than another."[2]

It is a common pastime of those with little talent to try to win points by attacking giants of the past. That is not the intent here. The contributions of Freud, Kinsey and others, whatever errors they may have made in their interpretations of female sexuality, will stand unchallenged and respected for years to come. But it is a disservice to deify a great individual to the degree that his or her work is not subject to review. Freud himself would have been displeased with this, as indicated by the comment he made in respect to his theories about sexuality: "On the other hand it should be made quite clear that the uncertainty of our speculation has been greatly increased by the necessity for borrowing from the science of biology. Biology is truly a land of unlimited possibilities. We may expect it to give us the most surprising information and we cannot guess what answers it will return in a few dozen years to the questions we have put to it. They may be of a kind which will blow away the whole of our artificial structure of hypotheses."[3]

The errors made in the past can be attributed largely to the fact that most of the investigators of female orgasm were men. Helena Wright, an English gynecologist, comments that: ". . . the thinkers and writers on the subject have been predominantly male, and all they can do is use their powers of observation and inquiry and interpret the results in comparison with their own experiences. It is lamentable that women have done so little thinking and writing on their own behalf and have accepted so meekly the passive role which men in western civilization have stamped upon female sexual interest."[4] Female orgasm has often been referred to as more subtle than male orgasm. In fact it is only more "subtle" because those male experts have never experienced it. William Masters and

Virginia Johnson, reversing a long-standing trend by studying sex from both the male and female viewpoints, proved in the laboratory that female orgasm is equal to, if not superior to, male orgasm. In clinical measurement the first two or three muscular contractions of the orgasm are quite intense for the male, probably to ensure the propulsion of the sperm toward fertilization. Although these initial contractions are more intense than the female's, the woman continues to have strong contractions—often up to eight or twelve—while the male contractions quickly decrease in intensity.[5] Masters and Johnson in their classic *Human Sexual Inadequacy,* wisely reflect: "Certainly, controlled laboratory experimentation in human sexual physiology has supported unequivocally the initial investigative premise that no man will ever fully understand woman's sexual function or dysfunction. What he does learn, he learns by personal observation and exposure, repute, or report, but if he is at all objective he will never be secure in his concepts because he can never experience orgasm as a woman."[6]

This point is a crucial one, for this lack of experience has led even giants such as Freud and Kinsey to make serious errors. As Aldous Huxley comments in *The Doors of Perception*: "By its very nature every embodied spirit is doomed to suffer and enjoy in solitude. Sensations, feelings, insights, fancies—all these are private and, except through symbols and at second hand, incommunicable. We can pool information about experiences, but never the experiences themselves."[7] Only as female experts begin to integrate their own experiences with recent scientific evidence will a clear picture about female orgasm begin to emerge from obscurity.

An excellent example of how the male lack of experience can cloud objective vision is seen in the incredible comments that two male "experts" made in the recent past about multiple orgasm in women. Edmund Bergler and William Kroger, commenting on Kinsey's work in their book *Kinsey's Myth of Female Sexuality*, remarked: "One of the most fantastic tales the female volunteers told Kinsey (who believed it) was that of multiple orgasm. Allegedly fourteen percent of these women claim to have experienced it. . . . Multiple orgasm is an exceptional experience. The fourteen percent of Kinsey's volunteers, all vaginally frigid, belonged obviously to the nymphomaniac type of frigidity where excitement mounts repeatedly without reaching a climax. . . . Not being familiar with this medical fact . . . Kinsey was taken in by the near-misses which these women represented as multiple orgasm."[8]

This "medical fact" put forth by these doctor has been totally repudiated by Masters and Johnson's scientific observations and physiological measurements. Indeed, for Kroger and Bergler and all other men, multiple orgasm is an "exceptional experience," but Masters and Johnson have demonstrated that it is a regular occurrence with many women and that probably all women have the potential to achieve multiple orgasm.[9]

Certain male writers have had such impact on the theories about female orgasm that they must be explored individually. The first of these is the father of modern psychiatry, Freud himself. In 1910 he stated: "If the woman finally submits to the sexual act, the clitoris becomes stimulated, and its role is to conduct the excitement to the adjacent genital parts; it acts here like a chip of pinewood which is utilized to set fire to the harder wood. It often takes some time before this transference is accomplished, and during this transition the young wife remains anesthetic. This anesthesia may become permanent if the clitoric zone refuses to give up its excitability, a condition brought on by profuse sexual activities in infantile life. . . .

If the transference of the erogenous excitability from the clitoris to the vaginal entrance succeeds, the woman then changes her leading zone for the future sexual activity.... The main determinants for the woman's preference for neurosis, especially for hysteria, lie in this change of the leading zone...."[19]

This classic statement, together with other inferences by Freud, was the genesis of the still raging controversy about clitoral versus vaginal orgasm. What is significant here, however, is that Freud and the psychoanalysts who followed indelibly established the idea that a woman who was unable to achieve orgasm or who had the "wrong" kind of orgasm was neurotic or mentally disturbed or, at best, "immature." This last judgment is based on the concept of the clitoris as an infantile source of pleasure, and in this view those women who persist in enjoying its stimulation have simply never matured. The supporters of these concepts are extensive.[11]

Even female disciples of Freud (who in light of recent evidence either must have been inorgasmic or chose to deny their own experience in favor of the theory as promulgated by the master) have often accepted this position. Marie Robinson, a psychoanalyst, in her popular book *The Power of Sexual Surrender* characterizes women who insist on stimulating their clitoris for sexual satisfaction as frigid and "masculine." Choosing theory over the weight of evidence from women she had seen, she asserts: "However, millions of women find this earlier method of gratification so satisfying that they are not motivated to move up to the mature level."[12]

It is important first to dispel this myth of the connection between female orgasmic difficulties and neurotic disorders. Fisher, after reviewing twenty-eight separate studies involving thousands of women, concludes: "But it is quite impressive that orgasm rate, which has often been regarded as one of the most basic indices of sexual responsiveness in women, does not differentiate psychotic and neurotic persons from those without gross psychiatric symptomatology.... A particularly striking discovery that was made was that a woman's ability to be sexually responsive is not related to how psychologically 'healthy' or 'unhealthy' she is. ... Contrary to psychoanalytic theory, it cannot be said that a woman's sexual responsiveness is an index of her emotional maturity or stability."[13] Mary Jane Sherfey, a female psychiatrist, after reviewing the findings of Masters and Johnson and modern embryology in her *The Nature and Evolution of Female Sexuality*, asserts: "With this understanding of evolutionary and embryological development, one conclusion must force itself upon psychiatric theory: *to reduce clitoral eroticism to the level of psychopathology because the clitoris is an innately masculine organ or the original libido is masculine in nature must now be considered a travesty of the facts*."[14]

It is important to comment on the actual issue of clitoral versus vaginal orgasm. Masters and Johnson's research demonstrated how modern biology has fulfilled Freud's prophecy that it might "blow away the whole of our artificial structure of hypothesis."[15] It offers the most impressive scientific evidence demonstrating the importance of the clitoris in the adult woman. The authors have shown that regardless of the source of stimulation, whether it is the clitoris, the vagina, or even the breasts, during orgasm the anatomical and physiological processes that occur involve both the vagina and the clitoris. They conclude with carefully chosen words: "There may be great variation in duration and intensity of orgasmic experience, varying from individual to individual and within the same woman from time to time. However, when any woman experiences orgasmic response to effective sexual stimulation, the vagina and clitoris react in consistent physiologic pattern. Thus, clitoral and vaginal orgasms are not separate biologic entities."[16]

Masters and Johnson further cite their finding that the clitoris is very important in promoting orgasm during intercourse. They observed that the thrusting action of the penis exerts traction on the vaginal outlet, specifically the minor labia, and this traction causes the hood or covering of the clitoris to move back and forth, thereby stimulating the sensory nerves of the head of the clitoris itself.[17]

Unfortunately, Sherfey and others have drawn the conclusion from this evidence of clitoral importance that the vagina is unimportant in female sexual response. Sherfey calls the clitoris ". . . the most important, and, in by far the majority of instances, the indispensable initiator of the orgasmic reaction."[18] Other less scientific but more emphatic observers, especially some of the leaders of the modern feminist movement, have also used Masters and Johnson's information to declare this position of "clitoral supremacy."

Indeed, millions of women received long-needed validation by the reinstatement of the clitoris as an integral part of adult female response. But, regretfully, this shift toward clitoral supremacy created a new group of supposed "female deviants"—those who insisted that in fact they *did* experience a vaginal orgasm and that it felt different from a clitorally stimulated one.

Unfortunately, Masters and Johnson may have aided this misinterpretation. In *Human Sexual Response* they appear to have slighted the very important work of the late Arnold Kegel, M.D., a gynecologist at the University of Southern California. Although Dr. Kegel's paper "Sexual Functions of the Pubococcygeus Muscle" is included in the list of references, the pubococcygeus muscle itself is not listed in the index, nor is its importance underscored

in the text. Instead, Masters and Johnson continuously
point to the existence of an "orgasmic platform" that develops in the mucosa or wall of the outer portion of the
vagina due to increased vasocongestion. In their discussion of orgasm it is the contractions of the "orgasmic platform" that are emphasized, and only cursory mention is
given to the contractions of the circumvaginal muscle
which underlies the mucosa.[19] The difficulty created by
their emphasis on the vaginal mucosa is that proponents
of clitoral supremacy used this as further proof of the in-
significance of the vagina as a source of sexual stimulation.

It is true that the vaginal mucosa or the walls of the vagina have very few nerve endings,[20] and that they are essentially insensitive (Sherfey devotes an entire chapter to
"Supplemental Data on Vaginal Insensitivity"). But, as
Kegel notes, there is a more than sufficient number of
sensory nerve endings in the pubococcygeus muscle that
underlies the vaginal mucosa. Helen Kaplan, a physician,
psychiatrist and sexual therapist and head of the Sex
Therapy and Education Program at the Payne-Whitney
Clinic of Cornell–New York Hospital, has also observed:
"... the deeper tissues do contain proprioceptive and
stretch sensory endings, especially in the outer one-third.
Contraction, palpation, distention and deep pressure, especially ... near the entrance and outer one-third of the
vagina, are reported as highly pleasurable and erotic by
many women. These pleasurable sensations produced by
vaginal stimulation differ in quality from the sensations
experienced when the clitoris is stimulated."[21]

In spite of all the confusion, it is possible to use the findings of modern biology, together with subjective reports
of female experience to bring clarity to this issue.

It may be helpful here to review the medical model of a
sensory-motor-reflex loop such as a knee-jerk reflex in

connection with female orgasm. A reflex has two separate components; the sensory component, which is the component that *receives* the stimulation, and the motor component, which is the muscular component that *reacts* to that stimulation. With female orgasm, the same motor component (muscular reaction) occurs in the circumvaginal muscle regardless of the source of stimulation. However, *experientially,* the way the orgasm feels to the woman having it depends on the source of the sensory input. Based on this difference in feeling, it is possible to distinguish the following three direct responses: the orgasm involving only direct clitoral stimulation with nothing inserted in the vagina; the orgasm that occurs with intercourse or with some penis substitute moving in the vagina *and* simultaneous stimulation of the clitoris; and the orgasm that occurs with intercourse or vaginal stimulation without simultaneous direct stimulation of the clitoris. But, to repeat: irrespective of the source of stimulation, the motor component of the orgasm always occurs in the circumvaginal muscle.

Kaplan, commenting on this, notes that the same separation of sensory and motor components of orgasm occurs in the male, but it has not produced the same controversy that has arisen surrounding female orgasm. In the male, it is the head and the shaft of the penis that receive the stimulation. As previously mentioned, these structures come from the same embryological source as the clitoris. But the *motor component* (the actual muscular contractions that expel the ejaculate) occurs in the muscles of the perineum and the base of the penis.[22]

Even Kaplan, however, indicates that the clitoris is probably the primary area of stimulation.[23] In regard to intercourse, this has yet to be determined. In the first place, Kegel's work shows that orgasm with coitus *can* be achieved more readily if the pubococcygeus muscle is in good physical condition (see Part 3, Chapter 1). More significantly, female patients at the clinic report that even without direct clitoral stimulation during intercourse, they feel enough sensation in the vagina to promote orgasm— if the muscle is in good physical condition. Furthermore, these patients report no sensation in the clitoris itself during intercourse. It is significant that these reports are from women who are able to achieve orgasm by directly stimulating their own clitoris during masturbation and are quite familiar with what clitoral stimulation feels like.

Finally, there exists a common condition in which the clitoris is tightly adhered to the foreskin. Sherfey, noting the importance of the traction on the foreskin for stimulation of the clitoris during intercourse, states emphatically that these adhesions would preclude orgasm with coitus.[24] Yet in a study at the clinic of 289 women with clitoral foreskin adhesions, many women had severe adhesions, such that only fifty percent or less of the glans could be seen on inspection, and they nevertheless achieved orgasm with coitus. If the clitoris is the primary source of sensation during intercourse, then it is difficult to explain coital orgasms in women with severe clitoral adhesions. It would seem, then, that although the clitoris is always involved in the attainment of orgasm, the current information does not allow the conclusion that it is the primary source of stimulation in intercourse. In fact, there is strong evidence to suggest that with intercourse the pubococcygeus muscle is the primary source of stimulation.[25]

This evidence does not suggest the sole primacy of the vagina or a reinstatement of the Freudian concept of "vaginal orgasm." And it most definitely does not suggest that a woman incapable of vaginal sensations is neurotic or immature. But it does demonstrate that the correction of a *physical* weakness of the pubococcygeus muscle, which is common, increases sensation and promotes coital orgasm in many women.

In any case, it is an exercise in futility to compare orgasms. No orgasm is better, more right, or more mature than another. Each should simply be enjoyed for itself.

Next to the confusion about the role of the clitoris in female sexuality, the greatest misconceptions concern the frequency of female orgasm. The Kinsey book on female sexuality, *Sexual Behavior in the Human Female,* was co-authored by three other men—Wardell Pomeroy, Clyde Martin and Paul Gebhard. Kinsey's data on who was doing what and with whom and when they were doing it provides an important description of the sexual patterns of males and females in America. However, his figures on the number of women achieving orgasm must be seriously questioned, as well as those of other known studies. Prior to and even subsequent to Kinsey, most of the studies were based on questionnaires sent to various groups.[26] As Kinsey points out, it is very difficult to determine the quality of the reply on a questionnaire. He felt that his study, which was done by personal interview, was much more accurate. He carefully stressed the study's ability to detect a reply that was faked or dishonest. Indeed, for most of the material presented, these factors did much to guarantee the quality of the information gathered. In the area of female orgasm, however, there are two major sources of error that essentially invalidate the data on this subject.

The first has to do with a woman's self-knowledge of the experience of orgasm. As observed earlier, women frequently come to the clinic with the express problem of having difficulty achieving orgasm with intercourse. On thorough questioning by a *female* interviewer, who often must describe how an orgasm feels to a woman, it often develops that in fact they have never had an orgasm at all. Many of these women are later seen in therapy and subsequently have their first complete orgasm. None of these women are intentionally lying. No cross-checking for honesty would have shown that these women were in fact non-orgasmic. They simply did not realize this fact themselves until the interview.

This finding has been observed by others.[27] Donald Hastings, M.D., in his book *A Doctor Speaks on Sexual Expression in Marriage,* relates: "Not uncommonly, when asked by a physician, a woman will express doubt that she has ever experienced orgasm and will ask the physician to describe it so that she can decide."[28] And Sherfey states: "Many women seem innocently vague and uncertain when we ask them to describe the nature of their sexual sensations, or they sound like a marriage-manual recitation on the nature of the orgasm. One wonders if this well-known difficulty women have in reporting their sexual sensations does not stem from the fact that they deceive themselves and us about the nature of these feelings—because they are afraid that what they *do* feel is not what they *should* feel."[29] It is important to note that this uncertainty is not apparent until a woman is asked to describe her orgasm. The need to have an orgasm to be sexually accepted is so great that many women suppress their own doubts and have thoroughly convinced themselves that they are orgasmic. Having no standard to compare with, they remain sure until asked to give specific details about their orgasm.

Kinsey's list of questions does not include a description of orgasm. Although in some cases he may have asked for details, his own opinion was that it was impossible to describe: "Some and perhaps most persons may become momentarily unconscious at the moment of orgasm, and some may remain unconscious or only vaguely aware of reality throughout. . . . Consequently, few persons realize how they behave at and immediately after orgasm, and they are quite incapable of describing their experiences in any informative way."[30] But, as Hastings puts it: "It is extremely unlikely that a woman who has actually experienced orgasm would be in doubt, just as it would be difficult to imagine that a man could be in doubt whether he had experienced the feelings of orgasm and ejaculation. Hence one usually considers that the woman who expresses doubt has never had an orgasm."[31]

Kinsey's second major source of error is even more significant. As Kinsey himself says: "In general, it is difficult to explore effectively unless one has some understanding of the sort of thing that he is likely to find."[32] It is apparent that Kinsey and his male collaborators, never having had a female orgasm, simply did not know what it was. They remark: "The fact that some women experience vaginal spasms or convulsions may provide some basis for the references in the psychiatric literature to a 'vaginal orgasm.' These vaginal spasms are, however, simply an extension of the spasms which may involve the whole body after orgasm.

"While the vaginal contractions may prove a source of considerable pleasure both for the female and for her male partner, it is a more difficult matter to determine whether the lack of vaginal spasms represents any loss of pleasure for a female."[33]

But as we have seen, the vaginal contractions are the orgasm. Without them the orgasm has not occurred.

In attempting to understand this misunderstanding of the physiology of female orgasm, it is interesting to note that although Kinsey's bibliography is one of the most extensive ever assembled, it does not include the important work of Kegel, which was published in 1952, one year before the publication of *Sexual Behavior in the Human Female*.

On the basis of all of the above, without disputing the many important findings of the Kinsey study, it must be concluded that the figures reported by Kinsey on the frequency of female orgasm in American women are invalid. Other, more recent sudies, such as Morton Hunt's *Sexual Behavior in the Seventies* published in 1974, give no reason to believe that they do not suffer from the same inadequacies.[84] Hunt's study was done by questionnaire, and there is no indication that a description of orgasm was elicted or used in tabulating the data given.

One other specific work should be mentioned briefly. Hailed by the publisher as the next logical step in the sequence started by Kinsey and Masters and Johnson, Seymour Fisher's *The Female Orgasm* is over five hundred pages in length and contains over a quarter of a million words and more than three thousand references. In spite of the book's length and its extensive and excellent review of the literature concerning female orgasm, its conclusions also must be seriously questioned.

Following his review Fisher devotes the majority of the book to a presentation of his own research and the conclusions drawn from that research. Admitting that his numbers are quite small, Fisher defends his study by claiming to have been more interested in the quality of the response a woman had than in the frequency of orgasm. He then gives ten excerpts from the descriptions of arousal and orgasm which he assures the reader were "chosen so as to constitute a representative cross section of the descriptions that were collected." Of these ten examples of the population Fisher was using to study female orgasm, not one seems clearly orgasmic by her own description. Not one description specifically mentions vaginal contractions. In fact, more of the histories contain statements that, based on the histories obtained in the clinic, provide a clear suspicion that the narrator is indeed non-orgasmic. For example: "Orgasm for me usually involves getting more and more tense until there is a final release, and then it drops down slowly. Actually, I wish that release were more violent at times."[35]

Of the previously mentioned patients at the clinic who subsequently discover that they never have had an orgasm, many describe their orgasm as a "release." This is usually the only description the woman has ever heard about orgasm, so when she feels her pleasure mounting and then it stops, the cessation of stimulation is often interpreted as the expected release. Many of these women, such as the one quoted above, have a vague suspicion that they are missing something.

In summary, although there has been no lack of information on the subject of sex in general and female orgasm in specific, much of what has been written contains serious error. One of the major reasons for the inaccuracies is that only in the last twenty years has medicine been free to examine the actual anatomy and physiology of sexual response without great fear of public censure. Indeed, as recently as 1930, T. H. Van de Velde, M.D., wrote in his introduction to his classic marriage manual, *Ideal Marriage*: "This book will state many things which would otherwise remain unsaid. Therefore it will have many unpleasant results for me. I know this, for I have gradually attained to some knowledge of my fellow human beings and of their habit of condemning what is unusual and unconventional. ... There is need of this knowledge; there is too much suffering endured which might well be avoided, too much joy untasted which could enhance life's worth. ..."[36]

The limitations imposed on scientific research hampered both Freud and Kinsey and probably led to some of the errors cited above. In his book, *Kinsey and the Institute for Sex Research*, Pomeroy, commenting on the little-known fact that the Kinsey team observed individuals actually involved in sexual acts, relates: "We observed directly more human sexual responses than any other scientists before Masters and Johnson. Later, the St. Louis team showed that on some points we were simply wrong, and they recorded many observations we missed. ... Looking back on this phase of our research, limited as it was, I can see that we were not more successful simply because we were far too anxious and cautious about what we were doing. ..."[87] Kinsey was afraid that if this aspect of his work were publicized he might be prevented from completing his monumental survey.[88]

Fortunately, Masters and Johnson have taken a huge stride toward reversing this long-standing difficulty. They have rightfully demonstrated the importance of having both male and female observers, functioning at equal levels, so that an accurate picture of sexual response can be elicited. Others, such as Helen Kaplan, are following the path opened by Masters and Johnson and using experiential material together with objective scientific evidence and bringing clarity to some of the long-obscured issues surrounding female orgasm. In the remainder of this text the work of these pioneers, together with the information learned from more than one thousand patients seen at the clinic, will be used to attempt to produce a clear picture of the actual causes of female orgasmic dysfunction and provide a suggested self-help program for eradicating this problem.

CHAPTER 3

Sex and Orgasm as Learned Behaviors

One of the major blocks in the path of those seeking help for their sexual complaints is the mystique of "natural-ness" that surrounds sexual response. Too often a woman looking for answers from her friend will be rebuffed by a statement such as: "Why, John and I never have to talk about sex; it just comes naturally." Sex has been described as the world's most popular competitive sport. However, it has one very important difference from all other competitive sports: you never get to see your competitors in action; you just hear about their track records—after the fact.

Unfortunately, such comments tend to create even further anxiety for the unfortunate woman who has never discovered the "natural" way to have an orgasm. It is important to explore just what truth there is to the widely held belief that sexual behavior is an instinct for animals and humans alike.

One reason given for this theory is that sex is important for the survival of the species and therefore must be an instinct. Examples of animals in heat and various mating behaviors are cited in defense of this position. Yet modern sex research has cast grave doubts on these suppositions even in regard to animals.

Harry Harlow, in his famous experiments with rhesus monkeys, separated some of the monkeys from the rest of the colony at a very early age. These isolated males and females were denied the early learning opportunities that other monkeys have. When as adults they were allowed to rejoin the rest of the group, they were incapable of any form of sexual functioning. They persisted in attempting awkward positions and failed to achieve actual intercourse. These monkeys showed symptoms of so-called impotence and frigidity, even though they were coupled with other monkeys who had been raised normally and were sexually experienced. Furthermore, these problems were irreversible in spite of later attempts at learning.[1] Similar experiments with wolves did demonstrate the ability of isolated animals to learn appropriate behavior after rejoining the community.[2]

Most sexual therapists have seen more than a few examples of couples who have been married for several years and have never actually accomplished penetration. Often patients show up at infertility clinics with histories of having intercourse with the penis moving in between the thighs but not actually entering the vagina.

Admittedly these are dramatic exceptions, and in fact the average person does reach adulthood with enough information to accomplish intercourse. But even this basic information is learned. What is less basic, and is even more unquestionably a learned phenomenon, is not "how to," but "how to enjoy" the sex act. Steven Neiger, M.D., a distinguished expert in human sexuality, has stated: "What nature has given us is the sexual *drive*, a longing for physical contact. What it has *not* given us is the wisdom and the knowledge of what to do with that drive. . . . The human sexual act cannot be performed unless a complex process of learning has taken place, especially if the sex act is to be enjoyable for both partners."[8]

Everybody must learn how to get the most out of his sexual functioning. However, as we shall see, most of what is learned is incorrect and often detracts from rather than enhances sexual enjoyment.

A very important part of the learning process is the development of a sexual role, i.e., what is appropriate behavior for a "boy/man" or a "girl/woman." In understanding sex-role development it should be recognized that boys and girls begin life with physically different bodies and that these physical differences evoke "girl versus boy" labels from the people in their lives, beginning in earliest infancy, when girls often get pink clothes and boys blue ones. From the moment of birth, teaching begins about what is appropriate behavior for boys and girls. As Marion Meade has written: "The double standard begins in the nursery; the real trouble is that it doesn't end there. Long after babyhood paraphernalia is outgrown, invisible pink and blue blankets continue to affect adult behavior. Nowhere is that more apparent than in the area of sexuality where inequality between the sexes makes for serious problems."[4]

While little boys are being molded to be stoic, assertive, and independent, little girls are taught to become ladies. Boys are instructed to "be tough; act like a man." Girls are protected and sheltered. Boys play rough-and-tumble games, have a lot of body contact, and are pushed into leadership positions. Girls begin to learn the roles appropriate to future mothers and homemakers. Deviations from the appropriate path are tolerated for a while, but if the excursion is too lengthy, it is not long before labels such as "sissy" and "tomboy" are attached to the straying child, often causing an emotional scar that lasts a lifetime.

John Money of Johns Hopkins University, a noted expert in the field of human sexuality and gender identity, provides dramatic documentation of the importance of early learning on the development of sex role-identity. In *Man and Woman, Boy and Girl* he presents a case history of an extremely unusual situation in which two identical twin male children were born; one of the twins suffered a surgical catastrophe at seven months when his penis was amputated accidentally during a circumcision operation done under electrocautery. Money relates how the distraught parents were convinced that the best remedy for this terrible problem would be to perform plastic surgery and create a vagina—in other words, surgically to change the boy into a girl. This was done at twenty-one months, and the child's name, clothing, hair style, etc., were changed accordingly.

Money quotes excerpts from an incredible diary kept for the doctors by the mother of these children. It offers dramatic proof of the influence a parent can have on boy-girl behavior:

"I started dressing her not in dresses but, you know, little pink slacks and frilly blouses . . . and letting her hair grow. . . . She likes for me to wipe her face. She doesn't like to be dirty, and yet my son is quite different. I can't wash his face for anything. . . . She seems to be daintier. Maybe it's because I encourage it. . . . One thing that really amazes is that she is so feminine. I've never seen a little girl so neat and tidy as she can be when she wants to be. . . . She is very proud of herself when she puts on a new dress, or I set her hair. She just loves to have her hair set; she could sit under the dryer all day long. . . ."

Money pointed out how the children's choice of toys reflected their assumption of their future sex roles. The girl asked for and was given dolls, doll houses, and the like, while the boy got cars, a gas station, and other typical male toys. By age five, the girl talked of growing up to be a doctor or a teacher and the boy a policeman or a fireman. At last follow-up, it was impossible to distinguish the little girl from other little girls of her age.[5]

Training for sexual response or lack of it also begins in early childhood. Women are encouraged to be dependent and passive in relation to men and to expect men to be sexually aggressive. As Meade states: "Even fairy tales ... serve as training manuals for female behavior. Sleeping Beauty waits until a brave Prince awakens her. Cinderella, leaving her slipper at the ball, sits at home and waits for her Prince to find her."[6]

Our modern-day Cinderella follows her lead. It is a young girl's role to wait anxiously at home while the boy calls at his convenience and makes the date. Even more significant for her future sexual response, or rather lack of response, are the encouragements and rewards a young girl receives for turning off her developing sexual impulses.

A growing girl represses her budding sexual excitement in response to society's demands and loses an important chance to integrate those feelings into her developing personality. She is allowed and even encouraged to experience the concepts of romance unconnected with any physical expression except perhaps a chaste kiss or embrace.

Throughout the dating years, a young girl acts as the policewoman and removes the probing hand from her dress, reminding her ardent lover that they must "wait until later"—until they are going steady, until they are in love, until they are engaged or married. The "until" varies, but the pattern is the same. The social rewards go to the girls who follow the rules:

B. B. was a fifty-two-year-old female seen at the clinic

for difficulty in achieving an orgasm with intercourse. Born the only daughter of a small-town minister, she related how she was extremely popular in high school and was an honor student and vice-president of her class. She carefully avoided associating with those girls who had bad reputations and was a favored child in the community. She learned accidentally to masturbate to orgasm by rubbing against her bed, and carried on this secret activity throughout high school despite tremendous feelings of shame and guilt. "I was very careful on dates, though, and never let a boy even touch my breasts. I knew if I gave in at all, my reputation would be gone."

Conditioning such as this sets up a pattern in which sexual excitement is wrong at all times but especially so with a man. Later this woman married a prominent banker in the community. Through twenty-five years of marriage, during which she gave birth to three children, she never experienced orgasm with her husband.

The following story was told by P. B., a twenty-nine-year-old legal secretary seen at the clinic for orgasmic dysfunction:

"I remember clearly being at the Junior Prom with Johnny. He was a very popular athlete, and I was proud to be at the dance with him. When we were dancing a close dance, I could feel his body next to mine, and I could feel the excitement and warmth begin to rise in me. There I was in my crisp white formal, corsage and all, in front of all those people, getting excited just like a tramp. I remember having to grit my teeth and force myself to regain control. I knew that nice girls don't allow themselves to feel that way or they'll get into trouble. By the end of the dance I was back to normal and was able to fend off Johnny's advances, as usual, when we made out afterwards."

The significance of this restraint is that it sets up a

conditioned reflex to hold back sexual feelings. Since it is a negative thing for young women to be sexually aroused, their holding back is accompanied by a reduction in anxiety, which in turn reinforces them in holding back these feelings. Eventually this becomes automatic, with repression the response to arousal. Years later these women have to be given help in recognizing that tight control over sexual feelings isn't "normal." They need to learn how to accept their own natural feelings and urges and how to respond to them.

Even straying from the path holds no promise of success for the young girl, for the burdens of guilt are carried with her. S. B., twenty-two, a beautician, was seen for a complaint of pain with intercourse:

"I left home when I was seventeen because I couldn't stand the restrictions placed on me by my parents. I had a rough time but managed to get a part-time job and go to beauty school. My virginity was gone before I left home, and I slept around with a lot of guys. But somehow I just never enjoyed it. I kept hoping it would get better, but it only got worse. And all the time I had this feeling burning in my gut that I was doing something wrong."

One of the most confusing things that a young girl must adjust to is the contradictions in the role that she is supposed to play. As she matures she is taught how to be aggressively seductive and alluring, while at the same time remaining subtle and passive. She is informed that her place in life will be dependent on her ability to attract and hold a man. She wears short skirts that reveal her legs, or long clinging ones; transparent blouses; bras that emphasize her sexuality, or no bra; and even lacy panties that no one is supposed to see but which help make her feel sexy. And yet when the eager young boy accepts the bait, she is often surprised and hurt. T. T., thirty-six, seen for the inability to achieve an orgasm recalled:

"After the party we parked and began our usual kissing, and suddenly he grabbed my breast. Of course I objected, and he became angry. He accused me of being a 'prick teaser' and said that I wore my low-cut blouse just to lure him on. I didn't understand what he was saying and broke into tears. He took me home and I never went out with him again."

Dishonest seductiveness is part of the degrading way women are taught they must behave to get what they want. Unfortunately, when they discover that they don't get it, the only answer to their misery is to seduce another man. M. A. came into the clinic because she was unable to have an orgasm with her husband. Her appearance and voice were immature and coquettish. She reacted in a very seductive manner toward her husband and toward the male therapist of the team they were seeing. Although she was a virgin when they married, she had learned to masturbate to orgasm as a child. She approached marriage confident that she would quickly be orgasmic, but in ten years of marriage she had failed to experience orgasm. In frustration, she had tried three extramarital affairs in quick succession in an attempt to find a man who would give her an orgasm. After that unsuccessful detour, she sought and received help and, with an understanding of her problem, began to relate differently to the men in her life, sexually and non-sexually.

A woman's comfort with her own and her partner's nudity also plays a significant role in the ability to relax and enjoy sexual pleasure. Once again women are short-changed in the development of these feelings. G. M. related: "In junior high school there were three private showers and a huge room with many showers together on the wall. The first girls in from PE always grabbed private showers. No one ever used the big shower room. As we were dressing, we all held our blouses over ourselves until we had our underwear on." Meanwhile the boys were in the adjoining gym showering together, making obscene comments and becoming comfortable with their own nudity.

The fashion industry picks up on this childhood conditioning and translates it into adult reality. Female fashions show just enough to provoke interest but of course never the whole body that lies beneath. Women develop an image of beauty that includes the bikini and uplift bra as an actual part of their bodies and regard the naked body as unattractive and even repulsive. The only part of their sexual anatomy that women are socialized to regard as attractive are breasts, but even there most women feel they fall short of the popular ideal. Their own are never as large or as small as they "should" be, never as high or as firm. So although a woman has a conscious awareness of her breasts, this awareness is usually negative. The genitals are relegated to "down there" and thought of as something dirty and strictly to be avoided if they are thought of at all. In contrast, men are conscious of their penises from early childhood on and are socialized to respect and even glorify their sexual organ.

But perhaps the most devastating part of the message that women are taught is that they must be beautiful and young to be sexy—not beautiful in relation to themselves, but rather beautiful in relation to other women and the accepted societal standards of beauty. A woman struggles to be beautiful not for herself but to catch a desirable man whom otherwise some other woman would get. She slims, covers her blemishes, paints her lips, polishes her nails, curls her hair, puts on false eyelashes, and dresses tastefully but seductively. Then she compares how she looks with the way other women around her look. If she compares favorably in her own eyes and in those of others, she considers herself sexually attractive. But stripped of her beauty aids and her clothes, her face and body naked before a lover, the average female feels inferior and insecure. Even the most attractive women are unsure of their beauty because of their concerns over a few extra pounds or lines or veins.

A woman's role is to look sexy so that the man gets excited from looking at her and does things to her that turn her on. But if she is less than sexy in her own eyes, she will have difficulty feeling relaxed and secure enough to be aroused.

J. B. was a thirty-two-year-old married woman who at the time she came to the clinic had never had an enjoyable sex experience in ten years of marriage. She reported, "Each time we would go to bed, I would undress in the bathroom and make sure the lights were out before I climbed into bed. Roger always told me he found me attractive, but after three kids and with stretch marks and flabby hips I just felt ugly. Actually I never did feel attractive, even when I was younger. With the right clothes and makeup I look pretty good, but without the props I don't have much to brag about."

Part of the concept of beauty is youth, connoting firm, smooth skin. It is toward this end that women spend billions of dollars a year on vitamins, exercise classes, hormone creams, beauty salons, cosmetic surgery. Women know they must look young in order to be attractive, so they make every effort to "stay" young and pursue the concept of youth. They think of themselves as young, they never tell anyone their age, and they are referred to as "girls." There are damaging effects from this elusive pursuit of youth, the most significant of which is that women think of themselves as immature, incapable and childlike. Children are not responsible for themselves; they wait to be taken care of. And this is exactly what women do sexually—wait for men to take care of them.

Another destructive message that women learn is the idealized concept of the role of wife and mother. Every women is raised to be "his" wife and the mother of "his" children, rather than to be herself. Built into the image of wife- and motherhood is purity, wholesomeness, and propriety. A basic dichotomy is established between a wife and a woman who likes sex.

This image of what is "proper" for a wife and mother can have a devastating effect on a woman's sexual response. The following is an example of a typical problem encountered at the clinic:

G. T. and I. T. came into the clinic after two years of marriage. They reported that they had lived together for six months before marriage. Sex at that time was spontaneous and delightful. Both of them felt that they were deeply in love, and they decided to get married.

Their sexual problems began on the honeymoon. Mrs. T. dressed up in a lovely white nightgown and went to bed. "For the first time in our relationship I felt inhibited. I just couldn't get aroused." This problem continued and grew gradually worse until the time the couple presented themselves for therapy. Although Mrs. T. had had orgasms before her marriage, at the time they were first seen she had not had one orgasm for two years.

Sexual history revealed that she had had a strict Catholic upbringing and held very puritanical views about marriage and the role of a wife. She had been able to suppress her feelings while living "illicitly" with her lover, partly because feeling sexy was what she was supposed to do in order to "get her man," but once having assumed the mantle of wife, she was no longer able to feel sexually free. Sexual therapy was oriented toward helping her understand her conditioning and giving her "permission" to be sexual. She was encouraged to compare her images of an ideal wife with those of her husband and was surprised to learn they were quite different. A thorough re-examination of the roles both had fallen into allowed her to rediscover her sexuality and regain her ability to have an orgasm. This loss or decrease of sexual enjoyment following marriage or the birth of a child is an extremely common occurrence.

Ironically, as Mary Jane Sherfey suggests, this sanctified image of women was created as a compensation for the suppression of their tremendous sex drive.[7] In a provocative theory, Sherfey suggests that when cultural evolution reached the point of a settled agricultural community, it became necessary to create a rationale for female monogamy in order that property rights could pass from father to son without confusion. The elevation of woman to a chaste status and the sanctification of that role accomplished this socioeconomic goal with much greater success than chastity belts and other forms of physical enforcement. But the price women pay for their honored position is too high. They learn to be good wives and mothers but not lovers. And while they stay home and raise the kids, their husbands are often out with secretaries who make great sex partners. This goes on until the secretary finds a husband, and then she becomes the wife and another woman becomes the lover.

Society, parents, and peers encourage a seductive, flirtatious, but basically asexual and controlled role during the developing years for the female, and this negative conditioning process, with its subtle reinforcement of the reward of "being a good girl," robs women of their basic biological birthright to orgasm.

Equally important to what is *learned* not to do is what is *not* learned. As adolescents, women are not encouraged to learn what an orgasm is or feels like. What they sometimes do learn is to be aroused. Kissing and petting are allowed; therefore a female often identifies the end point of sex as arousal and even accepts that as orgasm. R. B., a twenty-six-year-old woman seen with her impotent husband, related:

"Before I had therapy and learned to have an orgasm, I often felt hot, and it was always fun. I really didn't know I was missing anything, because I had no idea what an orgasm felt like."

Even more basic, females do not learn how to masturbate. Masturbation is the training ground for orgasm, and most girls simply do not learn until they are adults. Boys, in contrast, learn how to masturbate early. According to the Kinsey data, between the ages of sixteen and twenty, eighty-eight percent of males are masturbating, while only one-third of females are masturbating. This is significant in that masturbation provided the very first orgasm for sixty-eight percent of young males; starting after first ejaculation, ninety-nine percent of males go on to experience regular orgasm.[8]

Boys evidently share information about masturbation more readily. Kinsey noted that twenty-eight percent of his male sample learned to masturbate by themselves, but that seventy-five percent of the men had learned about masturbation before they actually began doing it.[9] But of women he reports: ". . . in the great majority of instances females learn to masturbate, both in pre-adolescent and later years, by discovering the possibilities of such activity entirely on their own." After elaborating on how most of the men began their masturbation prior to or shortly after the onset of adolescence, Kinsey says: ". . . most of them knew about masturbation and had actually been masturbating for ten or twenty years before some of their mothers and teachers even learned that there was such a phenomenon."[10]

As a consequence of this, Kinsey showed that boys simply learn at an earlier age than girls to be sexually responsive. His statistics showed that during early adolescence ninety-five percent of the boys experienced orgasm on the average of 2.3 times per week, but only twenty-two percent of the girls of like age were reaching orgasm. By late teens, ninety-nine percent of the males were having orgasms, while almost half of the females had not even reached their first orgasm. Kinsey concludes: "With this relatively limited background of experience and limited understanding of the nature and significance and desirability of orgasm, it is not surprising to find that a goodly number of married females never or rarely reach orgasm in their marital coitus."[11]

Another thing women fail to learn that is essential to sexual functioning is to be assertive. Woman's enculturated passivity affects her general behavior and specifically leaves her unprepared to take an active part in her own sexual response. Sexual feelings are engendered by movement of, for example, the hand against the genitals or the circumvaginal muscle against the penis. If a woman doesn't move her body in such a way that it feels good to her, if she depends on the male's movements to stimulate her to orgasm, her chances of reaching orgasm are reduced.

Again, the training learned in masturbation provides the goal and technique that, together with the willingness to move the body in search of stimulation, will produce orgasm.

B. S. was a twenty-nine-year-old male seen for secondary impotence. In therapy he revealed that his first sexual encounter was with a prostitute. "I remember that this apartment building manager where I was a lifeguard set it up for me. It was somewhat scary, but I tried to play it cool. After we undressed she put my penis in her and I just lay still on top of her. I just didn't have any idea that you were supposed to move. Then she started moving, and I recognized the feelings getting going just like when I did myself. I started moving in and out and was soon able to climax."

Obviously women who have never learned to masturbate and have not achieved orgasm cannot know what it feels like. Lacking this knowledge, they do not pursue the goal of orgasm during intercourse in the same way as someone who is more familiar with the feelings being sought. Furthermore, again unlike men, they lack the social permission to pursue the goal in the first place.

One reason suggested for this difference in society's approach to male and female orgasm is the notion that the male orgasm is more important because ejaculation is imperative for propagation of the species. This is true, but it does not justify the conclusion, held by many, that a man's sexual response is more natural than a woman's. As we noted earlier, the similarities in the anatomy and physiology of male and female sexual response far outweigh the differences. It seems unlikely, then, that one sex with anatomy and physiology similar to the other's would, in a cultural vacuum, learn "spontaneously" while the other did not.

The study of cultures other than our own bears this out. Not all cultures specifically discourage female response and encourage male response. In fact, in some areas of the world the opposite is true, as Robert J. Maxwell pointed out: "What evidence we do have suggests that it is sometimes the woman's orgasm, rather than the man's, that is the primary concern in coitus. This seems to be true, for example, among the Crow Indians of the American plains, the Mangaians of Polynesia, and the Trukese of the Caroline Islands, where a man may be ridiculed if he reaches orgasm before his partner. In fact for the Trukese, female sexuality is so much more of a dominant interest that . . . 'in contrast to our own society, it is for the Trukese the vagina rather than the penis which is the primary symbol of sexuality.' "[12]

Other cultures specifically react to any attempt on the part of the female to attain sexual pleasure, as Ronald Deutsch reports: "The Chiricahua tribe deals with the problem by disallowing it, holding that women should display no emotions in the sex act. The Colorado Indians and such primitive cultures as that of the Lepcha insist that the woman remain entirely passive, thus making her pleasure unlikely."[13]

In 1949, the noted anthropologist Margaret Mead stated in her classic *Male and Female*: ". . . the human female's capacity for orgasm is to be viewed much more as a potentiality that may or may not be developed by a given culture. . . ."[14]

Her observation reflects clearly one of the important principles underlined in this book: that orgasm, like sex, is a learned behavior. Some women learn it; most do not. Most men learn it; some do not. It is the culture or society in which a man or a woman is raised that dictates to an incredible degree whether or not that individual will subsequently become orgasmic.[15]

The impact of society can be shown by a comparison with the culturally deprived minority child who has a reading problem. Without the same learning opportunities, parental encouragement, career goal and possibilities, peer example, etc., the poor black simply doesn't learn as well as the suburban white. Yet when cultural issues are eliminated on intelligence testing, the basic intelligence is often very similar.

Males not wishing to add to their "white man's burden" of guilt by recognizing this deprivation in learning potential will be embarrassed or antagonistic to this concept. Nevertheless, the evidence is clear that women are the victims of a society which does not actively encourage their pursuit of sexual satisfaction.

Any woman can learn, yet most do not. Fortunately sexual therapy, applying the principles of behavior therapy and learning theory, has begun to help significant numbers of women eradicate this early learning deficit with "adult education." The remainder of this book will provide a self-help program that uses the principles and techniques developed in clinical practice.

PART 3

The Solution

CHAPTER 1

Physical Barriers to Sexual Functioning

There are two separate steps involved in the learning of any new task. The first is to see that your "equipment" is in good working order, and the second is to learn how to use that equipment. This is true both of mechanical tasks, such as carpentry, and for more physical endeavors such as learning to ride a bicycle—or learning to have an orgasm. This chapter will discuss some of the physical problems women may have that can act as barriers to healthy sexual functioning and how these problems can be successfully treated. Once your body is functioning properly, the task of learning how to have an orgasm can be accomplished with greater ease.

The subsequent chapters in this book will deal with a step-by-step program for achieving orgasm. This chapter is an important prerequisite to that program. Your chances of success will be seriously affected if you do not first read this chapter and involve yourself in those parts that are applicable to you.

You must be in good physical condition. An athlete, for example, undergoes extensive medical examinations and physical training before he or she begins to compete. Training is often tedious and boring, and sometimes the trainee wonders what the exercises have to do with his or her goal. A young high school football player who has yet to play his first game grumbles considerably about pushups and training practice and wonders what pushups have to do with football. But when he is trying to outdistance a pack of pursuing players to the goal line, he understands the importance of good conditioning.

You too may become bored with the process of getting yourself in proper physical condition, especially if you have never had an orgasm and are very much interested in getting on with the business of learning how. Fortunately, the parts of this chapter that will apply to the majority of readers can be done at the same time they are beginning the learning program.

PUBOCOCCYGEUS DEFICIENCIES:

Arnold Kegel, M.D., a gynecologist at the University of Southern California, discovered that dysfunction of the pelvis musculature causes urinary stress incontinence (a common condition in which the woman loses urine when she coughs or sneezes). He began to seek a non-surgical treatment for this condition and developed a method of teaching women to contract the vaginal muscle by using a passive-resistant device attached to a biofeedback mechanism—the Perineometer.[1] Patients were taught to tone this muscle so that the pubococcygeus became a firm, straight platform providing strong support to the pelvic organs. As a result of working with thousands of patients, he accidentally discovered that vaginal sensation, which increased as a direct result of doing these exercises, allowed many women who had previously not felt anything during intercourse to develop sensation and achieve orgasm. He observed: "Whenever the perivaginal musculature is well developed ... sexual complaints are few or transient. On the other hand, in women with a thin, weak pubococcygeus muscle ... expressions of indifference or dissatisfaction regarding sexual activity were frequently encountered. When a more careful history was taken, the symptoms revealed a definite pattern. ... In the patient's own words: 'I just don't feel anything'; or 'I don't like the feeling'; or 'the feeling is disagreeable.' ... Following restoration of function of the pubococcygeus muscle, numerous patients incidentally volunteered the information: 'I can feel more sexually'; and some experienced orgasm for the first time."[2]

It is one of the mysteries of the history of sexual therapy that although "Kegel's exercises" are known and practiced throughout the world for the treatment of stress incontinence, the sexual aspects of this work have been largely ignored, even by such noted investigators as Kinsey and Masters and Johnson.

As noted earlier, the pubococcygeus muscle is one of the supportive circumvaginal muscles and, as such, aids in holding the pelvic organs in the proper position. Unfortunately, in many women the condition of the pubococcygeus muscle is poor, resulting in a lack of sensation during intercourse which prevents the possibility of orgasmic response. These women frequently complain of simply not feeling anything during intercourse. Kegel stated: "Every woman with sexual complaints should be investigated for possible dysfunction of the pubococcygeus muscle. In a large percentage of cases it will be found that 'lack of vaginal feeling' and so-called frigidity can be traced to faulty development of function of the pubococcygeus muscle."[3]

Kegel presented the case history of a forty-two-year-old woman who had been married twenty-one years. When first seen she had been suffering for seven years from a frequent loss of urine. A physical examination revealed poor condition of the vaginal muscle. The patient did not know how to contract this muscle. She was placed on an exercise program which was successful in treating her urinary problem. Kegel related that at the final visit the patient revealed that the exercise program had dramatically improved her and her husband's sex life together. A further history revealed that although both had wanted more sex, intercourse had not been enjoyable and so had occurred infrequently. Following the restoration of her muscle—undertaken because of the urinary problem—the couple had intercourse several times a week and the patient was able to achieve orgasm, which previously she had not been able to do. Kegel reported that two years later the couple were still having good sexual relations.[4]

Although Kegel reintroduced the significance of the pubococcygeus to the modern medical world, the importance of this vaginal muscle has been recognized in other cultures for centuries, although usually in terms of producing pleasure for the male. Alex Comfort quotes the Indian *Anagaranga*, written in the sixteenth century: "She must ever strive to close and constrict the Yonī [vagina] until she holds the Lingam [penis], as with a finger, opening and shutting at her pleasure, and finally acting as the hand of the Go-pala-girl, who milks the cow. This can be learned only by long practice, and especially by throwing the will into the part affected.... Her husband will then value her ... for the most beautiful ... queen in the three worlds. So lovely and pleasant to the man is she-who-constricts."[5]

Ronald Deutsch states in *The Key to Feminine Response in Marriage*: "Some primitive and oriental people have observed the need for such muscular control and strength and teach young women accordingly. In one African tribe, no girl may marry until she is able to exert strong pressure with the vaginal muscles."[6]

Even in the United States prior to Kegel, early pioneers in the area of sexual dysfunction recognized the significance of poor condition of the pubococcygeus muscle, although their presentations were not nearly so scientific or so extensive as Kegel's. At the beginning of this century, both R. L. Dickinson, the physician to whom Masters and Johnson give great credit for development of the knowledge of sexual physiology,[7] and T. H. Van de Velde, in his *Ideal Marriage*, published in 1926, noted that after women learned to use their vaginal muscle, sexual functioning was enhanced.[8]

Poor condition of the pubococcygeus muscle apparently exists in many women, regardless of whether or not they have had children. However, the natural consequences of vaginal delivery as well as some surgical procedures performed by physicians can worsen the condition of the muscle. As Kegel observed: "In the past, loss of sexual feeling following childbirth has often been explained on the assumption that the wife's affections had been transferred from the husband to the child. Actually, many women fail to recover muscular tone after the trauma of childbirth."[9]

As an example, Kegel relates the case history of a woman who married at twenty-two. For two years sex was good, but after the first child it deteriorated. Following the birth of a second child the couple separated several times. The woman explained that intercourse had become unpleasant and so was avoided. She stated that she had lost feeling during intercourse. Examination showed a thin, atrophic pubococcygeus muscle. According to Kegel, the patient was placed on an exercise program. "After six weeks husband and wife stated that sexual feeling had returned. Three years later, the couple reported that sexual relations continued as gratifying as prior to the birth of the first child."[10]

Not uncommonly, as a baby's head is being delivered, the doctor will perform an incision known as an episiotomy. J. Oliven, M.D., states in his textbook *Sexual Hygiene and Pathology*: "Mediolateral episiotomy . . . tends to cause major damage to the pubococcygeal muscle on one side. . . . Such an unrepaired muscle appears to be a major contribution to unsatisfactory sexual function. . . ."[11] Fortunately these childbirth traumas also repsond to an exercise program.

The vaginal portion of the pubococcygeus muscle is important in a woman's sexual function, since, as we have said, the muscle underlying the vaginal walls is well supplied with proprioceptive, or pressure-sensitive, nerve endings. This allows the woman to feel a great deal of sensation when firm pressure is applied against this muscle; during intercourse, pressure against the muscle is increased when the woman deliberately contracts the muscle against the penis.

A determination of the condition of the pubococcygeus muscle can only be made by a detailed examination, one which can be performed by any gynecologist and is often part of a standard pelvic exam. This should consist of a careful digital exam of the entire muscle body in both a contracted and a relaxed state, as well as a measurement of the strength and control of the muscle with a Perineometer device. There is no way that a woman can examine and diagnose the condition of her own muscle.

The Perineometer was designed by Dr. Kegel so that a doctor could measure the strength and control of the vaginal muscle. It also functions as a passive-resistant device to be used in exercising the muscle. Exercise against passive resistance is the best way to strengthen any muscle in the body. By lifting weights, you use passive resistance to strengthen the biceps in your arms. The resistance in this case is the weight, but it is passive because it moves upward as pressure is exerted against it by the arms of the person lifting it. The Perineometer functions in the same way for the vaginal muscle. The resistance is the device inserted into the vagina, but it is passive because it deflates (moves) as pressure is exerted against it by the contraction of the vaginal muscle.

As the vaginal tube deflates, the needle on the gauge rises in direct correlation to the amount of pressure brought about by the contraction of the muscle, so you can tell to what extent you are squeezing the muscle. As the vaginal muscle relaxes, the needle on the gauge lowers back to its starting position. This way women who have no control over their muscle can discover what they must do to make the needle rise. To those women who do know how to contract the muscle, the biofeedback device shows how much they are squeezing. This is important, because with something inserted into the vagina, there is much less awareness of movement with contraction than when there is nothing in the vagina. (This explains why the vaginal contractions with orgasm during intercourse feel more subtle in comparison to the distinct contractions from solely clitoral stimulation.) Women who are doing maintenance or corrective exercises without the Perineometer do not need a biofeedback device, because they can easily feel the vaginal muscle moving with each contraction.

Four factors are important in evaluating the pubococcygeus muscle: control, strength, tone, and atrophy.

Control of the muscle is the woman's ability to contract it (squeeze it together) and the ability to hold it in a contracted state. Poor control is evidenced by the lack of ability to hold the contraction evenly to a count of ten seconds. Although this indicates a need for corrective exercises, they may be done without the Perineometer. The exercises described in Part 3, Chapter 2, Step 2 can be done as corrective exercises for this type of muscle deficiency, but they should be done for a period of twenty minutes a day until adequate control of the muscle is gained, and then should be reduced to the maintenance level of five minutes a day indefinitely.

Strength is the degree to which a woman can contract the muscle. Poor strength is diagnosed when the actual amount of the contraction is very little as measured on the Perineometer. Poor strength of the pubococcygeus requires corrective exercises with the Perineometer.

Tone is the way the muscle feels on examination. Poor tone is diagnosed when the muscle is broad, but instead of being firm to the touch it is mushy and stringy, either all the way around or in parts, and has a poor degree of resistance.

Correction of poor tone requires the use of a Perineometer and usually takes approximately three months of exercising.

Atrophy of the pubococcygeus muscle is varied in its presentation, but essentially it indicates that the muscle is underdeveloped. In some cases, there is a narrow ligamentous band outlining the pubococcygeus muscle around either edge, but the muscle body itself between these bands is missing. These ligamentous bands are generally very strong, and a woman with this type of muscle atrophy will usually register a high reading on the Perineometer. Corrective exercises take a considerable period of time, perhaps months or more, until the entire missing body of muscle is regenerated and becomes firm to the touch. In some women segments of the muscle are missing, usually from a developmentally unhealthy muscle which has undergone trauma during childbirth or pelvic surgery. In many cases muscle tone and function can be completely repaired by corrective exercises, but the time required varies according to the severity of the damage. In addition, cystocoele (lack of bladder support, which causes the bladder to fall against the front vaginal wall) and rectocoele (lack of rectal support, which causes the rectum to fall against the back vaginal wall) can often be corrected through these exercises instead of expensive surgical repair. Correction of muscle atrophy always requires the use of the passive-resistant device, the Perineometer.

If upon examination it is determined that the pubococcygeus muscle is broad, firm, and completely intact all the way around the vagina, and the strength and control are good, then no corrective exercise need be done, although maintenance exercises should be instituted and continued throughout life (see Part 3, Chapter 2, Step 2).

Use of the Perineometer:

If you are going to use the Perineometer, there are a few things you should know first. Since the vagina is not an open tube, but rather a collapsed, potential space, insertion of the Perineometer will create a certain amount of pressure on the gauge even without contraction of the muscle. This can be referred to as the "resting" reading. Upon contraction of the vagina, the needle will rise to a peak and go no further; this can be referred to as the "squeezing" reading. A woman who is doing the exercises should record both the resting and the squeezing figures each time she does the exercises and should give this information to her doctor for his evaluation. Supplied with the Perineometer is a booklet with graph paper which provides a place for this written record.

Care of the instrument is simple—but, to avoid infection, don't lend it to anyone else. All you need to do is wash the part that goes into the vagina, using a wet but not dripping washcloth and taking care not to get water underneath any of the rubber parts. Then dry it and store it in a clean, airtight place, such as a plastic bag sealed with a clothespin or a rubber band. The tube should be disconnected at the glass connector to allow the vaginal tube to remain fully inflated. Before using, simply reconnect the tubing, making sure that the vaginal tube is first filled with air.

Sometimes the vaginal tube of the Perineometer develops a leak and the tube fails to inflate after being squeezed. This part can be replaced separately by the manufacturer, as can all the parts of the device. The most expensive part is the gauge, which will break if it is dropped or knocked against a piece of furniture, so treat it carefully.

The Perineometer is available only by a physician's prescription. Although there are some popularly advertised products on the market which purport to have the same function as the Perineometer, there is no other device available anywhere that has any effect at all on measuring or strengthening the vaginal muscle, or changing the tone of the muscle. Do not be misled by dishonest advertising into buying something that cannot help you. The Perineometer is the only device designed by Dr. Kegel and the only device proved in medical studies to be beneficial to the vaginal muscle. If another credible device does become available, your doctor will be able to tell you about it. If he or she is unable to find any information about it, you can assume that it is a waste of your money.

The use of the Perineometer must be supervised by a physician, and changes in the pubococcygeus muscle must be evaluated by periodic examination.

Exercise Instructions:

Lie flat on your back (you may use a small pillow under your head for support) with your legs in a frog position (knees bent, soles of feet together). Insert the vaginal tube into the vagina (you may use some K-Y Jelly for lubricant if you feel you need it, but under no circumstances use Vaseline or baby oil—they will destroy the rubber). Try to relax your abdominal and vaginal muscles. Then, visualizing the two sides of your vagina, bring those two sides together in a squeeze, as if you were clapping your hands together. At the same time, you will be squeezing as if you were trying to stop urinating, except that you must not squeeze your abdominal muscles; you will also be squeezing as if you were trying to stop a bowel movement, except that you must not squeeze your buttocks. You will be squeezing only the part at the bottom, not at the front and back. *The exercises must be done to a count of six seconds:*

1: squeeze slowly and deliberately;

2: hold steady;

3: continue to hold steady;

4: continue to hold steady;

5: extra squeeze, even though you think you are already squeezing as much as you can (you *may* use your abdominal muscles to help you with this squeeze);

6: relax the muscle fully before doing the next squeeze. Count to yourself: one thousand one, one thousand two, etc., until you reach six. These corrective exercises must be done for a minimum of twenty minutes daily in order to achieve results, and are best done for twenty minutes twice a day. Depending on the condition of your muscle, your doctor may want you to do them even more frequently.

In addition to the instructions above, you should also do exercises with urination. As you sit on the toilet, spread your knees wide and rest all of your weight on your forearms against the tops of your thighs. (This prevents your abdominal muscles from having to support you in a sitting position, thus allowing them to relax so that you do not contract them when you contract your vaginal muscle.) As you begin to urinate, instead of letting the urine out all at once as you normally do, let it out only a small squirt at a time (about a teaspoon). Then stop the flow of urine for a moment and let out another squirt. Continue doing this until your bladder is empty. Do this each time you urinate, until you can do it easily and have perfect control over your urination. Then you can discontinue this part of the exercises. The purpose of the urination exercises is to aid you in gaining control of the pubococcygeus muscle, control which you need in order to exercise it properly. The urination exercises have no effect on tone or strength of the muscle.

Some women experience a "nervous" feeling when they contract the vaginal muscle. This is not an emotional problem but a physical one. It is caused by trying to move a weak, flabby muscle that isn't used to moving; it will disappear as the tone of the pubococcygeus muscle begins to improve, usually in two or three weeks.

Many women become discouraged after doing the exercises for a short time because they don't see any difference on the gauge from when they first started. This does not mean that the muscle is not improving. Many times, especially when the strength is fairly good to begin with, the exercises are directly affecting the tone of the muscle rather than the strength, so that improvement and progress are being made but are not showing up on the gauge. It for this reason that a woman needs to be under supervision of her physician, so that she can receive frequent periodic examination and evaluation of the pubococcygeus muscle.

Some women become discouraged because they are not able to squeeze to any significant degree, or to hold the squeeze for the duration of the exercise. However, the exercises should be done, or at least attempted, whether or not the woman is successful at them. This attempt will have positive results on the muscle, and with time and practice the woman will gain strength and control. For example, if a woman squeezes but can hold the squeeze steady for only one second instead of the three seconds recommended, she should still *try* for three seconds, even if the needle on the gauge is falling. In other words, she should make the effort as instructed, even if the results of that effort are not what they should be. In the long run the results of the exercises will be evident, and they will be positive.

PROBLEMS WITH CONTRACEPTION:

The development of reliable birth control methods has had an overwhelming effect on the female sexual response. There is little doubt among women—regardless of the pro and con arguments of male psychologists—that fear of pregnancy is a serious deterrent to the enjoyment of sex. Textbooks are filled with examples of women who did not begin to enjoy sex until after menopause, when the risk was over.[12] Reliable birth control for women who don't want to conceive is a *must* for full sexual response.

Unfortunately, the problem does not end there. The issue of choosing a contraceptive device, as well as evaluating its positive and negative effects on the body and on sexuality, is a complicated one. In our limited space we cannot give complete information about the various con-

traceptive devices. The following is only a commentary on
the effects of some of them on sexual response.

The birth control pill is the most commonly used contraceptive device. No clear picture has been drawn on the
possible negative effects the pill may have on female sexual response. In 1970 Malcolm Potts, M.D., Medical
Director of International Planned Parenthood, reported
that it was very difficult to assess sexual response because
of the difficulty in quantifying it. He also noted that another variable to be considered was that a woman's sexual
response varies with age and from woman to woman. In
the first report on Enovid, Pincus noted that coital frequency, which of course is not necessarily in direct relation to libido, rose in fifty percent of the women and fell
in forty percent.[18]

According to Alan Guttmacher, M.D., President of
Planned Prarenthood Federation of America:

"The majority of patients when first on the pill seem to
enjoy intercourse more, perhaps largely because they are
freed from fear of pregnancy. . . . As time goes on, few
patients have a genuine increase in libido and few a genuine reduction." Later he states more directly that those
women who do experience a decrease in libido should try
a different pill or consider sequential pills.[14]

Dr. Francis Kane of Tulane University reports depression, lethargy, and loss of sexual interest in women on
oral contraceptives.[15] He has been quoted as saying that
for every woman who experiences an increase in sex drive
when on the pill, ten or more experience a decrease. And
LeMon Clark, M.D., has said:

". . . the strongest objection, first brought to my attention in a personal communication from Dr. William Masters some two years ago—but since that time confirmed at
least ten or twelve times in my own practice—is that pro-
longed use of the pills, that is two to four years, may

bring about an almost complete loss of libido or sex desire...."[16]

Clark, among others, advises: "Any young woman taking the pill for birth control should very promptly turn to another method if she finds herself developing any loss of sex desire."[17] Barbara Seaman, in her book *Free and Female*, points up the problem with this comment: "With time, an experienced woman whose sex drive declines on the pill is usually able to figure out why, and she stops taking it. Inexperienced women have no base level of comparison."[18]

In summary, the pill can and does increase sex drive and the ability to achieve orgasm for some women. Women who have experienced a change for the worse in their sexual functioning and women who have never enjoyed sex or who are just beginning to have sexual experiences should weigh this with other factors in choosing their method of birth control.

The other most commonly used contraceptive agent is the intrauterine device (IUD). This device is placed inside the uterus and has no effect on the rest of the body or on the hormonal balance, as do the pills. It is probably the least complicated device to use, since, after insertion, essentially it may be forgotten. Like the pill, it does not require any interruption of lovemaking. About the only disadvantages reported are that occasionally the strings attached to the IUD have caused the male to experience discomfort, which, however, can usually be remedied by cutting the strings shorter or leaving them longer, depending on the difficulty; and secondly, in some women the IUD causes extra bleeding and cramps, and for these women it would probably interfere with sexual response, at least during menses.

It is important to note that besides the effect that contraceptives such as the pill or the IUD may have on sex, there are other considerations, such as side effects and potential hazards from their use. These issues have been much publicized and written about, and even medical authorities admit they do not have all the answers on the safety of these devices. Obviously, however, an unwanted pregnancy has serious emotional and physical side effects and hazards as well.

The condom, the diaphragm, and contraceptive foams and jellies are also still commonly used. In fact, women's groups concerned over the side effects of the pill and the IUD have begun to recommend a return to the diaphragm. Although the latter is somewhat less effective than the two most popular methods, it still has a high rate of pregnancy prevention, with usual estimates ranging around ninety percent if it is used properly. In regard to sexual functioning, the most common arguments against condoms, diaphragms, and contraceptive foams and jellies are that they are messy and unesthetic, that they interfere with manual or oral lovemaking, and that their use interrupts the sexual act or causes it to be premeditated and therefore unspontaneous. Clark, however, refutes the issue of "mess" in regard to the diaphragm. "The jelly or cream should be put above it, on the top of the depressed dome as it is inserted, not around the rim or below it, where it may make a gooey mess of the act of intercourse." More important, he suggests an alternative way of looking at the issue of interruption, both for the diaphragm and for the condom:

"Where women object to its use, I suggest that as part of sexual play they let their husbands insert the diaphragm. And I point out that fifty years ago when all we had was the condom—which men objected to ... I would tell them to stop thinking of themselves and to start thinking of their wives. By taking the very slight degree of trouble to use a condom, he was permitting his wife to relax and enjoy intercourse without fear of pregnancy; if he looked at it that way, instead of serving as a sexual depressant the use of the condom could serve as a sexual stimulant. The same argument, in reverse as it were, applies to a woman and the use of the diaphragm. . . . When it is properly fitted and the patient carefully instructed in its use, in my opinion it is still the best method we have."[19]

Alex Comfort in *The Joy of Sex* notes that some people complain of decreased sensation, but he goes on to encourage the treating of condoms and diaphragms as part of love play.[20] Indeed, one reason given for the failure rate of diaphragms is that women have difficulty with a method that causes them to actually handle their genitals. But men and women should be able to talk about their likes and dislikes during love play. The discussion and use of a diaphragm or condom can be made intimate instead of an embarassing interruption. It is true, however, that condoms—even the more expensive "skins"— do reduce sensation for the man, and some women also object to the way they feel to them.

Vasectomy of the male, in which the tubules in the scrotum are cut, has become much more popular of late. It does have the unfortunate emotional side effect of causing impotence in some men, but much can be done to prevent this by good counseling before surgery. Another potential drawback is that it is a permanent change rather than a reversible one.

Coitus interruptus, or withdrawal, constitutes an obvious interruption in lovemaking, and it is also so ineffective as a birth control measure that we do not recommend it.

The rhythm method does not allow you to make love when you want to, and it discourages sex at times of the month when some women are most easily aroused.

A book that is helpful in weighing the non-sexual aspects of choosing a birth control method is *Birth Control and Love* by Alan Guttmacher, written in 1970. It is an excellent summary by a medical doctor who is known worldwide for his expertise, fairness and humaneness.

Finally, however, the decision must be yours. Birth control is a very individual choice—one that each man and woman and each couple must decide for themselves. Listen to everyone else first, but listen finally to yourself in making your decision.

AGING AND HORMONE DEFICIENCY:

When a female ages, her ovaries stop functioning. This causes what is known as the menopause and includes the cessation of the monthly menstrual cycle. The accompanying symptoms vary from woman to woman, with some women having uncomfortable ones such as hot flashes. The ovaries secrete hormones, and it is the decrease or lack of these hormones—often called sex steroids—that is responsible for most of the symptoms. An almost universal change that may or may not cause problems is the change that occurs in the skin and secretions of the genitals.

Oliven discusses the specific effects of hormone deficiency on the female genitals:

"Gradually, the tissues of the *vulva* become thinner . . . and the introitus [opening] becomes increasingly constricted, i.e., 'tight' and inelastic. . . . The *vaginal mucosa* [wall] becomes atrophic in many cases; it may appear reddened and shiny, thinned and be somewhat tender. . . . Genital *secretions* become scant . . . general pelvic relaxation is common. . . . The regressive changes in the genitalia, even with increased artificial lubrication, may make the sexual act too uncomfortable to invite frequent repetition."[21]

Masters and Johnson have reported on the dramatic difference in the appearance of the vagina in women in their thirties from that of women in their sixties and seventies. They also report that many older females complain of pain following intercourse, especially intercourse that occurs infrequently or lasts a long time.[22]

The changes that occur can be extremely disturbing to the woman who is undergoing them. A dramatic example of hormone deficiency is illustrated by the following letter received at the clinic:

"Dear Doctor: I have had my uterus removed, but my ovaries are still there, and I am fifty-five years old. About a year ago, I started breaking out with painful blisters in the vaginal area. Then the skin in the area started changing color, first to white, then to black near the inner lips. Sex became more painful than before. Then one side of the inner lip began disappearing, along with a numbness, itching and aching, and the clitoris began to swell shut. Every time my husband and I had intercourse, the skin would develop small burning tears at the clitoris and the space between the vagina and the rectum, which caused me great pain. Meanwhile, the inner lip on the right side went away completely, and now the left side is three-quarters gone.

"I've been to three doctors, and they each tell me something different—a gynecologist, a surgeon, and a dermatologist. I don't know what to do and I'm getting desperate. I no longer enjoy sex with my husband because all I feel is burning and pain when he touches me. I'm afraid with my parts disappearing I'll turn into a man and this frightens me. Is what is happening to me normal? Will my pain go away when the other lip disappears completely? What can I do?"

Obviously the process of watching your sexual organs actually disappear is disquieting. J. B. was a fifty-five-year-old patient seen for lack of sexual arousal. Initial examination revealed no clitoris. Where there had been a clitoris, there was only a faint red line. Subsequent steroid replacement and minor surgical lysis of adhesions revealed that due to senile changes in the vulva, the tissues had closed over the clitoris, and this accounted for its "disappearance."

Following hormone replacement, a dramatic improvement occurred in the appearance of the genitals: the clitoris "reappeared," and with additional sexual therapy to overcome her anxieties, this patient became orgasmic with masturbation and intercourse.

Masters, whose early research was in this area, is a solid supporter of sex-steroid replacement. There is good medical evidence that the changes referred to above in the genital tissues can be prevented or reversed by adequate sex-steroid replacement.[23]

Others such as Clark question the wisdom of using steroids by pill or injection, when locally applied creams are effective and are more economical.

Also, as Masters and Johnson point out, many women pass through menopause without any need for steroid replacement. They claim that one important key for avoiding problems is a continuous level of sexual functioning. Not every woman, therefore, will need steroid replacement. Proper diet, a consistent sex life, and keeping active in general are good preventive medicine for all the effects of aging—including changes in the female genitalia. However, if the discomforts of hormone deficiency are interfering with your sexual functioning, hormone therapy—local or systemic—should be considered to help alleviate your discomfort and improve your ability to function normally.

CLITORAL ABNORMALITIES:

During the physical examination performed as a preliminary to sexual therapy at the clinic, one of the more frequent questions female patients ask is whether or not their clitoris is normal and in the right place. Many women have been told by their sex partners that there is something wrong with them. But Masters and Johnson, as a result of their extensive research, completely refute the concept that variation in size and position of the clitoris affects female sexual response.[24]

Clitoral foreskin adhesion, in which the foreskin or the prepuce of the clitoris becomes attached to the head or glans, is a condition found in many women. It occurs when small grains of smegma are trapped between the two skin surfaces. Rubbing on the clitoris becomes painful because of these buried particles of smegma that tend to act like grains of sand.

The significance of this clitoral foreskin adhesion for female sexual response is unclear. In a review of 411 female patients seen at the clinic, 279, or 79.1 percent, had adhesions; 33.6 percent of these were graded as severe, which meant that more than fifty percent of the glans was adhered to the foreskin.[25] This condition has also been called buried clitoris,[26] adherent prepuce[27] and clitoral phimosis.[28]

The research done at the clinic did not clearly demonstrate any negative effects from this condition. Many of the women with severe clitoral adhesions reported absolutely no difficulty achieving orgasm. Others with severe adhesions had never had an orgasm, and all variations between these extremes were found.

Wardell Pomeroy reports in his book *Kinsey and the Institute for Sex Research* that Kinsey noted the condition in some women and had the cooperation of a physician in lysing the adhesions. He felt that in several instances it had been quite helpful.

LeMon Clark also feels that the condition is clinically important. In *Advances in Sex Research* he reports seeing one hundred consecutive women of which ninety-two had clitoral adhesions. In seventy-five of these cases he felt that the adhesions were significant enough to interfere with normal sensation. He states strongly that these adhesions can have far-reaching effects on a woman's sex life.[29]

Mary Jane Sherfey also concludes that the condition is a block to adequate response: "Obviously, the adherent prepuce practically precludes the possibility of coital orgasms."[30]

Masters, however, is not convinced of the significance of this condition.[31] Oliven states that it is usually asymptomatic,[32] and other gynecologists deny its importance.[33] Virtually the only point agreed upon is that the condition exists. Further research will have to be done before its significance is known. Obviously, if clitoral foreskin adhesion is in fact unimportant, it reflects seriously on the value of clitoral stimulation during intercourse, since an adherent prepuce could not provide as much stimulation to the glans of the clitoris as one which was not adhered.

A similarly controversial issue is the concept of clitoral circumcision, i.e., surgical removal of the foreskin. W. C. Rathmann, M.D., reported in the *Journal of General Practice* on the results of female circumcision: "If cases are carefully selected, one should expect 85–90 percent to show satisfactory improvement." From this minor surgical procedure[34] Rathmann has claimed dramatic improvement in many marriages on the brink of divorce. Others disagree,[35] and Semmens has suggested that since Masters and Johnson's observations indicate that direct stimulation of the glans of the clitoris is not usually done because the glans is too sensitive, it follows that surgical removal of the foreskin is not likely to be helpful.[36] Further research is indicated before any factual statement can be made on the value of circumcision in the female.

PAINFUL INTERCOURSE:

This section will deal only with the known physical causes of pain. All too frequently a therapist assumes without examination of the patient that the pain she suffers is emotional. R. B., a twenty-nine-year-old librarian, was referred for examination after five months of psychotherapy for painful intercourse. Examination revealed an intact hymen. Digital stretching of the hymenal ring reproduced the pain she experienced during coitus. The vaginal muscle secondarily showed signs of vaginismus (spasm) as a reaction to the pain of stretching the hymen. Hymenotomy (surgical rupture of the hymen) was recommended and subsequently performed.

Emotional or psychological pain should only be presumed after a competent medical exam has ruled that physical problems are unlikely.

Painful intercourse from physical causes can be divided into superficial and deep pain. Superficial pain stems from problems at or around the vaginal opening. The above-mentioned intact hymen is one cause, as are inadequate hormonal levels of the vaginal walls as noted previously. Scars from childbirth, injury or episiotomies have been shown to cause pain in some instances.[37]

Persistent vaginal infections make sex unpleasant. The use of antibiotics and contraceptive pills has been frequently blamed for chronic infection. Rectal intercourse with subsequent vaginal penetration has been suggested as a cause of persistent vaginitis.[38]

Chronic vaginal or urinary infections can be the result

of repeated lack of orgasm. As mentioned earlier, pelvic vasocongestion occurring in the normal female provides the necessary vaginal lubrication for intercourse; however, frequent sexual excitement without orgasmic response leaves the pelvis congested with blood, and seepage of the lubrication continues well beyond its usefulness. This creates irritation and chafing and produces the signs and symptoms of infection. Urinating over this raw area causes burning and pain. Continued irritation provides an excellent breeding ground for infection. Not only the irritation but the sexual problem—the lack of orgasm—should be treated.

Lack of lubrication is one of the most common causes of superficial pelvic pain. Often this lack is more a result of lack of knowledge of sexual physiology than actual physical pathology. Lubrication begins seconds after the woman becomes aroused. If she is lying on her back, the vagina angles inward instead of up and down, and as the vaginal lubrication is produced, it pools at the inside end of the vagina rather than moving to the outside. And it is in this position (on her back) that most women are stimulated during love play. Either partner can "cure" this simply by using a finger to bring the ample lubrication to the surface. However, the real absence of lubrication *can* be a demonstration of a lack of sexual interest. The female lubrication is produced by the same basic physiological process as the male erection and is a sign of sexual excitement. If, however, in spite of interest, there is still no lubrication, artificial lubrication is both normal and sensible.

Deep pelvic pain has a number of causes. Included are lacerations of the broad ligaments supporting the uterus, endometriosis, ovarian cysts and tumors, infection in the ovarian tubes, and post-surgical adhesions. All these conditions require a pelvic examination for diagnosis.

Unfortunately, even a competent examination by a medical-sexual therapist often is not enough. As Masters and Johnson observed, some women have such negative experience with sex that they use the symptoms of pain to avoid it.[39] As more and more women are helped to enjoy sex and have orgasms, it is hoped that they will have no need for such escapes.

POOR HYGIENE:

Patients often ask about the importance of douching. As we noted earlier, women are brought up to think of sex and their genitals as dirty. The advertising and sales of feminine hygiene products is a multimillion-dollar industry.

Actually, unless your doctor specifically suggests it, douching is unnecessary and can be harmful. It can remove the protective bacteria that are naturally present in the vagina and allow an infection to begin.[40] The vagina has a normal cleansing action that moves any secretions or semen toward the outside. All that is required for adequate hygiene is to keep the outside labia and clitoral area clean, using soap and water. Inadequate hygiene can produce unpleasant odors and interfere with lovemaking, but frequent washing of the external genitalia will be sufficient to prevent any unpleasant odors. It may be necessary to retract the foreskin of the clitoris and, using a cotton swab or piece of gauze, remove any accumulation of smegma. Male genitals also need frequent washing, as females are no more "dirty" than men. If you experience difficulty in carefully cleaning your genitals, Step 1 in the next chapter will probably prove helpful.

POOR GENERAL HEALTH

It is important to conclude this chapter with a brief note about general physical condition. Every patient seen at the clinic is carefully questioned about general medical health, and any medical problems are treated before she begins sex therapy. Before you start the treatment program outlined here, we advice a general physical check-up by your doctor, as well as a careful exam by a physician who is knowledgeable in the field of sexual physiology.

Poor diet, excessive use of alcohol or drugs, and chronic fatigue are all serious blocks to sexual enjoyment. Alcohol and drugs, other than certain specific prescription items, are forbidden for patients at the clinic while they are in therapy. Cigarette smoking, possibly one of America's most serious addictions, also contributes to poor general health and should be discouraged. The seductive advertising that suggests sexual gratification to the person who smokes a certain brand of cigarettes never reveals the clear medical evidence which shows the toll that cigarettes take on heart, lungs, blood vessels, and other parts of the body.

CHAPTER 2

An Eleven-Step Program for
Achieving Self-Stimulated Orgasm

This chapter and the one following set out the step-by-step program we have developed and used to help women who have difficulty in achieving orgasm.

Basically, orgasmic dysfunction can be divided into two categories. The first includes the woman who has never achieved orgasm by any means. The second includes those women who have had orgasm, usually by masturbation, but who have rarely or never been able to achieve orgasm with a partner. The most common complaint of the latter group is the inability to climax during intercourse.[1] As we said earlier, these two problems are usually caused by lack of knowledge.

The concept of a step-by-step masturbation program for treating orgasmic dysfunction was first set forth by LoPiccolo in 1972 in the *Archives of Sexual Behavior*, where he reported one hundred percent success in treating fifteen cases of primary orgasmic dysfunction by this procedure.[2]

Before actually beginning the learning program, it is important to reread the description of orgasm in Part 1. It is easier to reach your goal if you know exactly what that goal is before you start.

The learning program has two parts: learning to have an orgasm by self-stimulation (masturbation), and learning to have an orgasm with your partner (manual stimution and intercourse). The women in both of these categories—those who have never had an orgasm and those who have, but not yet with a partner—should begin with this chapter. Even those women who can already masturbate to orgasm, will find reviewing this chapter helpful, especially Steps 2, 6, 8 and 11. *It must be emphasized that in this program, learning to masturbate to orgasm is a prerequisite to learning to be orgasmic with a partner.*

A woman must feel comfortable looking at and touching her own body if she is to feel at ease when her partner looks at and touches her body. A woman must be able to experience strong sexual feelings alone without shame or guilt in order to be comfortable experiencing those feelings with a partner.

Masturbation is a laboratory wherein a woman can learn about her own arousal and orgasm.[3] After all, masturbation is the way that men learn. A young boy will often have his first orgasm in a "wet dream," an ejaculation while he is asleep. But his first orgasm while he is awake, and indeed perhaps his first several hundred orgasms while he is awake, are almost always by masturbation. Once he is thoroughly experienced in how to move his hand over his penis or his penis against the bed in a way that reliably produces orgasm, he goes on to learn how to move his penis in the vagina in a way that will produce orgasm.

It is important first to discuss masturbation before proceeding, for as Helen Kaplan observes in *The New Sex Therapy*: "Not surprisingly, the instruction that the patient masturbate to reach orgasm often evokes considerable anxiety in patients who have been taught from childhood to regard masturbation as dangerous and shameful."[4]

The message about female masturbation is so strongly reinforced that few dare question it later on in life. But because it is possible for an adult to look more rationally at things, it is possible for an adult to unlearn that lesson. However, since there are so many myths about the harms of masturbation, it may be helpful to discuss them before proceeding.

"No other form of sexual activity has been more frequently discussed, more roundly condemned, and more universally practiced than masturbation."[5] As Morton Hunt observes in *Sexual Behavior in the Seventies,* "Even though any reasonably well informed single young man or woman knows that nearly every other single man or woman masturbates at least occasionally, almost no one will admit, even to an intimate friend, that he or she does so. . . . Not even lovers, in their most intimate confessions, tell each other that this is still part of their repertoire of sexual behavior."[6]

Historically, the teaching about masturbation has included prophecies of physical and/or mental illness and moral decadence. Kinsey, reviewing the literature about masturbation, noted that in orthodox Jewish codes it was considered a sin, and at times in Jewish history it was even penalized by death. Catholic religious codes also condemn it as a sin. Some of the women questioned by Kinsey believed that masturbation was the cause of many of their physical problems, including pimples, stomach upsets, poor posture, weak hearts, etc. He reports: "Many persons believe that masturbation may harm one physically."[7]

The suggestion that masturbation is the source of these problems is understandable if one reviews the statements made about masturbation by physicians in the past. In 1760 Tissot, a Swiss physician, published a very influential text, *L'Onanisme: Dissertation sur les Maladies Produites par la Masturbation.* He connected masturbation to epilepsy, feeble-mindedness, impotence, bladder ailments, convulsions, and paralysis.[8] Krafft-Ebing in his *Psychopathia Sexualis* connected it to sexual deviations and mental disorders. Brecher in his review *The Sex Researchers* notes, "Krafft-Ebing's *Psychopathia Sexualis* is still amazingly popular in bookstores and from mail-order houses. ... Some physicians still keep a copy of Krafft-Ebing on their shelves and refer to it on occasion. Two new editions were published in the United States in 1965. Both carried new introductions by reputable psychiatrists—introductions which casually conceded that perhaps Krafft-Ebing was a little out of date, but which failed to alert readers sufficiently to the deeply damaging nonsense (such as the alleged relation between childhood masturbation and lust, murder, and homosexuality) with which his pages are filled."[9]

Kinsey lists eighteen other "experts" who report on the physical damage caused by masturbation, some as recently as 1936. In fact Greenbank revealed that in 1961 a survey of five Philadelphia medical schools showed that: "... half of the students have a feeling that mental illness is frequently caused by masturbation. Even one faculty member in five still believes in this old, and now discredited idea."[10]

The book *Sexuality and Man,* put out by the prestigious Sex Information and Education Council of the United States, Inc. (SIECUS), contains the statement, "Medical opinion is generally agreed today that masturbation, no matter how frequently it is practiced, produces none of the harmful physical effects about which physicians warned in the past. The physical effects of masturbation are not significantly different from the physical effects of any other sexual activity."[11]

The more modern view of masturbation debunks the threats of damnation, disease, and degeneracy. But it does convey its own negative message, which goes something like this: "Masturbation is not evil and is nothing to panic about, provided it is not excessive." Unfortunately, it is never made clear just what is meant by excessive. Does it mean that it is all right to masturbate once a month, but not once a week? Or is it all right to masturbate once a week but not once a day? Or is three to ten times a day excessive? These vague warnings leave people feeling more worried about masturbation than does the obviously ridiculous claim that it causes insanity. Also integral to the modern view is the idea that masturbation is a form of sexual behavior that the "normal" person outgrows, causing every adult who masturbates (which is the majority of adults) to question his or her maturity.

Actual facts show that in Kinsey's era ninety-two percent of males and sixty-two percent of females masturbated. Hunt's statistics show almost identical figures for the seventies—ninety-four percent for males and sixty-three percent for females. Additionally, the females are doing it at a younger age and continuing to do it as they grow older. And most important, Hunt's data shows that seventy-two percent of husbands and sixty-eight percent of wives continue to masturbate after marriage.[12]

It is important to look at masturbation not as a stage one passes through but as a lifelong supplement to a normal sex life. It is an enjoyable experience, having the advantage that it does not require a partner, and one which is qualitatively different from lovemaking with a partner. Many people feel guilty about masturbating if there is the possibility of sex with a partner, an attitude which sets up masturbation as a poor second rather than as a valuable addition to a normal sex life. Ford and Beach reported that among sub-human primates masturbation is frequent in spite of the availability of receptive partners.[13]

In addition, a willingness on the part of both partners to masturbate is the only way that one can completely take the responsibility for his or her own sexual functioning, thus relieving the partner, when necessary, of the burden of responsibility. For better or worse, your orgasm is yours and not the property or responsibility of your partner. Aldous Huxley puts it poetically in *The Doors of Perception*: "Embraced, the lovers desperately try to fuse their insulated ecstasies into a single self-transcendence; in vain."[14] Your sexual response is locked within your own body. Even during intercourse, male and female remain separated by the skin of the penis and the lining of the vagina. Just as you taste and digest your own food, so must you take responsibility for your own orgasm.

Further, if both partners are able to masturbate freely with each other, it greatly increases sexual variety within the context of a relationship. As Alex Comfort says in *The Joy of Sex*: "A couple who can masturbate each other really skillfully can do anything else they like. Handwork is not a 'substitute' for vaginal intercourse but something quite different, giving a different type orgasm, and the orgasm one induces oneself is different again from orgasm induced by a partner. In full intercourse it is a preparation—to stiffen the man, or to give the woman one or more preliminary peaks before insertion. After intercourse it is the natural lead-in to a further round. Moreover, most men can get a second orgasm sooner from partner stimulation than from the vagina, and a third after that if they masturbate themselves. . . . However much sex you have, you will still need simple, own-hand masturbation—not only during periods of separation, but simply when you feel like another orgasm."[15]

Most important, as LoPiccolo has observed: ". . . since masturbation is the most probable method of producing an orgasm and since it produces the most intense orgasm, it logically seems to be the preferred treatment for enhancing orgasmic potential in inorgasmic women."[16]

The number of times you masturbate while you are learning how may be quite different from the number of times once you know how. When you are a student, you need to spend a lot of time studying. Once you know how to masturbate to orgasm, the frequency will depend solely on your desires. These desires vary from person to person. Some may masturbate once or twice a month, others once or twice a day, or more. All these patterns are perfectly normal. Each woman's frequency of masturbation will vary, depending on her mood, her general level of rest or fatigue or tension, her health, the monthly hormonal cyclic changes, whether she is pregnant or not, whether she has a partner, whether or not she can arrange for privacy, and the number of things she has to do in any given day.

When you learn how to masturbate gradually, you can deal with whatever anxieties you encounter along the way and overcome them before going on to learn more complex lovemaking. There is a basic premise that underlies this entire program: if some activity or behavior makes you anxious, the best way to get over it is to repeat the activity at least six times in ten days. In most cases, a person will start to feel more comfortable with the particular activity, and once this happens, the anxiety will continue to diminish with repetition. This is the type of behavioral therapy known as implosive therapy.[17]

For example, if at first you feel nervous looking at your genitals and perhaps think they are unattractive, do it every day, and by the sixth day it will probably feel easier than it did on the first day. And if you keep on looking every day after that, eventually you should feel completely comfortable about it, just as if you were looking at your arm. What this means is that in order to be able to feel totally comfortable doing certain things sexually, you need to be willing to experience small amounts of anxiety in order to overcome that anxiety.

P. A., a twenty-nine-year-old law student who was in therapy to learn to have an orgasm, told us: "Of course I've never looked at my genitals; why should I? All that my vagina means to me is smells, blood and babies, and none of that is pleasant!" She was advised to look at her genitals five times a week, and at the clinic two weeks later she recounted the following: "I'm so excited I can hardly stand it. I actually feel good looking at myself. Do you know that I'm even beginning to believe that my genitals are attractive? I never imagined that I'd ever feel that way. It was awful the first few days, but it got easier and easier to look, and then it was just like looking at any other part of me."

After all, that is exactly what your genitals are—another part of *you*. And you make the decision as to what to do with that part of your body. It is your right to arouse yourself if you wish, and nobody can take that right from you unless you let them. This may be difficult to believe, though, when for the first twenty years of your life you *knew* that touching yourself "down there" was very wrong.

In following the self-help instructions outlined in this book, it is very important to keep the following things in mind. First, you must take each step sequentially. This means that you should begin with Step 1, complete it according to directions before moving on to Step 2, and so on for each of the steps. This is true even for those women who already know how to do some of the steps.

In our practice the success rate is very poor for those women who do not follow the proper sequence of steps.

Completing a step means doing it either for the suggested period of time (e.g., two weeks) or for a shorter time if you reach orgasm first. The success of the program depends on your learning to do each step without feelings of anxiety, embarrassment, guilt or shame. Anxiety stifles sensation, which means that if you do not conquer your uncomfortable feelings about the simple step you are performing, you will not feel sensation at a more complex level. And without sensation, you will never have an orgasm.

If you follow the instructions for the specified period of time and are still experiencing anxiety, embarrassment, guilt or shame, do not go on to the next step. Repeat the exercise as instructed for as long as six weeks without moving on to the next step. If at the end of six weeks the levels of your negative feelings are reduced somewhat, continue the exercise for as long as it takes to feel fully comfortable.

There may be those who, even at the end of six weeks, do not experience any reduction of anxiety or guilt. Often simply doing sexual exercises brings back the memory of earlier painful experiences. Discussing your feelings with a sympathetic friend or lover can often help you uncover the source of your anxiety. But if these negative feelings persist, do not go on with the program. Instead, consider seeking professional help. A competent psychotherapist or sex therapist can be of great help in overcoming deep-seated sexual blocks. (For referral to a qualified psychotherapist or licensed sex therapist, call the nearest medical center, university-based medical school, or county medical society.)

If you follow the instructions for the specified period of time and simply do not experience any additional positive sensations or feelings of arousal, don't worry. Move on to the next step. The point of all these steps is to give you alternative ways of learning to have an orgasm. You may need to work through all of them before you are successful—in fact, this is true for many women in our practice.

It is important to realize that it took many years to *not* learn to have an orgasm. Most women who follow the program learn to have orgasms relatively quickly, but you should understand that it is not a one- or two-day procedure. Success with this program requires self-discipline, enthusiasm and dedication.

It may help you to know the average length of therapy for patients treated at our clinic. For a woman who has never had an orgasm at all, it takes approximately eight to twelve weeks to learn to masturbate to orgasm, either with her hand or with a vibrator. A woman who can masturbate to orgasm, but who has never had one with manual stimulation by her partner, usually takes approximately four weeks to learn how. And for the woman who is orgasmic with self- and partner stimulation, but not with intercourse, it takes approximately six to eight weeks to learn to be orgasmic with intercourse, provided that the pubococcygeus muscle is in reasonably good condition. All of these estimates apply not just to that particular period of time, but to the time spent actively working on the problem. The instructions in this book allow you a slightly longer period for learning.

Many women may find it difficult to follow the recommended time schedule. You may have guests in your home, you may go on vacation or a business trip, or you or someone in your family may become ill. Most women can withstand an interruption in the learning program of up to about six weeks, and can then simply resume the exercises where they left off. If resumption at the same place in the program is not successful, go back to the previous step; if that is not successful, then to the step before that. For your ease in following the program, there is a summary of steps after Step 11, but it should be used only after reading all of the steps in the text completely.

STEP 1 SELF-EXAMINATION

How: The first thing to do is to look at your genitals and learn to feel comfortable looking at them. Surprisingly enough, this first step is often the most difficult. If at all possible, see that you are alone in the house; otherwise arrange for privacy and lock the bedroom door. Take a hand mirror and lie down on the bed. Using the mirror, look carefully at all of the different parts of your genitals, as well as your breasts. Separate the labia (lips) and look at all the details. Find all the parts on the diagram (Figure 1, facing page 39) and find the same parts on your body. Pay particular attention to locating the three parts of the clitoris: the shaft (the tubelike structure just below the pubic hair which runs in an up-and-down direction—you can locate it by rolling your finger from side to side over it); the glans (the little pealike structure located between the shaft and the top of the labia minora); and the foreskin or prepuce (the movable hood or covering which overhangs the glans). Spend at least ten minutes on this entire process.

Repeat this exercise four or five times a week until you feel totally comfortable. You may consider this exercise completed when you can do it without feeling any anxiety, embarrassment, guilt, or shame, and when you can correctly identify each part of your anatomy. Take as long as six weeks to do this, and a minimum of one week.

Why: Most women feel that female genitals, their own included, are unpleasant and generally to be avoided. These feelings may stem from early confusion between the anus and vagina because of their similarity and proximity. As Fisher states: "Analysts have reported that in the fantasies of female patients in psychotherapeutic treatment, one finds a confusion between vagina and anus, with the result that 'dirty' attributes of anality become linked with the vagina."[18] Negative attitudes associated with menstruation and the use of such demeaning expressions as "on the rag" or "the curse" may also contribute. These early attitudes are fed by modern commercialism, especially the advertisements for feminine hygiene deodorants. However, learning to feel good about your genitals is not so difficult as it seems. All it requires is a little patience and a little time.

The reasoning behind Step 1 is that you must be able to feel totally comfortable simply looking at your own genitals before you can hope to feel at ease touching them. You must be familiar with your anatomy before you can use and enjoy it. Privacy is important so that you can be relaxed and comfortable doing the exercise.

STEP 2 PUBOCOCCYGEUS MUSCLE EXERCISES

How: These exercises will help increase the sexual sensation in your vagina. They should be done with nothing inserted in the vagina. You may do them lying down, sitting, or standing; essentially the same sensation will result. Visualize the two sides of your vagina. Try to bring these two sides together in a slow, steady squeeze, squeezing as if you were trying to stop urinating. Try to concentrate on the vagina, not the rectum, although the latter will contract somewhat on its own. If you are unfamiliar with how to move your vaginal muscle, practice with fast flicks at first instead of slow squeezes until you can feel what you are doing. (Note: The exercises as outlined in this step are designed not to correct any muscle deficiency but only to increase vaginal sensation and awareness, and to improve control. We suggest an examination by a gynecologist to determine the physical condition of the pubococcygeus muscle. If the muscle has poor strength or tone, skip this step and refer back to Part 3, Chapter 1.)

While you are contracting the vagina, you should not be contracting your abdomen. Placing one hand on your abdomen will remind you not to use the abdominal muscles. It is easier to keep the abdomen relaxed if you are standing or lying down instead of sitting. Doing the exercises properly requires a great deal of concentration, so don't talk, read, or watch television while you are doing them. Soft music is usually not distracting.

They should be done to a count of six seconds:

1: a slow, steady contraction of the vagina;

2: hold steady;

3. continue to hold steady;

4: continue to hold steady;

5: extra squeeze without first relaxing, even though you think you are already squeezing as hard as you can (you *may* use your abdominal muscles to help you at this point);

6: relax the muscle fully.

Then start the entire process over again. The easiest way is to count to yourself, "one thousand one, one thousand two," etc. Do this for five minutes three times during the day if possible; otherwise any combination of time that equals fifteen minutes.

This step is completed when you can easily squeeze

your muscle to the six-second count for fifteen minutes a day and when you do so you get at least a mild sexual feeling. It should feel good when you are doing it. When you've accomplished this, begin Step 3, but *continue doing the exercise for five minutes three times a day until you learn to have orgasms,* and then decrease to five minutes a day for the rest of your life.

Why: Exercising the pubococcygeus muscle is helpful in increasing sexual feeling and gaining an awareness of the muscle as a sexual organ. As noted earlier, the importance of the vaginal muscle has been known for centuries but primarily as a means of giving pleasure to the male. However, it can be very important to *your* enjoyment of sexual intercourse. The pubococcygeus muscle contains many proprioceptive (that is, sensory) nerve endings. When these nerves are stimulated by the movement of the penis or other object against the muscle, it is very pleasurable for the woman. By developing control of this muscle and using it to grasp the penis during intercourse, you will greatly increase your own sensation during coitus.

When you move any muscle, it is impossible to move only *part* of it; the entire muscle always moves at one time. The muscle that surrounds your vagina also surrounds the rectal and urinary areas. Thus, when you squeeze your vagina together, you feel the movement in the urinary and rectal areas as well.

When you are first learning to contract your vagina, it is all right to try fast flicking movements of the muscle instead of slow, deliberate squeezes, because this will give you a sense of just what you are supposed to be moving. But these fast flicks will do you little good in gaining control of the muscle, in generating sexual feelings, or in learning how to use the muscle during intercourse. They are only useful in helping you to identify the muscle and to begin learning to move it. Because the six-second count method has been found to be the most strenuous workout you can give the muscle, it also produces the greatest results.

In order to move the pubococcygeus muscle as much as possible, and to be able to feel it moving as a separate muscle, you must keep your abdominal muscles as relaxed as you can. Relaxation is the key to experiencing sexual feelings. It is important to be able to use your vaginal muscle without tensing elsewhere, such as in the abdomen or buttocks, because such tensing can cut off the flow of sexual feelings. (As the rectum partially contracts when you squeeze your vagina, there will be minimal tensing of the buttocks around the rectal area, which is unavoidable.)

It is necessary to allow your muscle to fully relax before beginning the next squeeze in order to get as much movement in the muscle as possible, and therefore the most exercise. If you do not fully relax it, it isn't moving as much as it could if you did relax it, and with less movement it is getting less exercise. And of course the relaxing part is the easiest, so give yourself the benefit of a short pause before starting to squeeze again.

Many women have difficulty learning to move the vaginal muscle adequately. During this initial practice period, a woman will often feel nervous when squeezing her muscle. This nervousness is not emotionally but *physically* induced. If you experience this, it is an indication of poor muscle tone and you should see your gynecologist. (See chapter entitled "Physical Barriers to Sexual Functioning.")

A woman who has a healthy muscle may feel anxious in general about the idea of focusing attention on her vagina. She may worry about what she will do if she doesn't experience any difference in sensation. This kind of anxiety is related not to the actual doing of the exercises, but to her concern over her success or failure. Any new undertaking is a possible source of anxiety, and certainly this is true of changes involving one's sexuality.

Although many women will feel anxious over the possibility of failing to learn to have orgasms, some will feel anxious over the possibility of succeeding. The latter stems from an uncertainty as to how being orgasmic will change you or your personality. Although these fears are very real, it is important for you to know that it is normal to have orgasms and that becoming orgasmic does not change a woman's basic personality. Some women fear that it will increase their sexual desires to an unmanageable extent. This is not the case. What usually occurs instead is an increased feeling of self-worth and self-confidence. The best way to deal with your anxiety is to share your feelings with a close friend or lover.

That these exercises can be helpful to you as you proceed with the rest of the program is shown by the following example. L. M., a fifty-one-year-old housewife who was seen in therapy recounted: "One of the things that helped me to feel sexy while I was learning to masturbate successfully was doing my vaginal exercises. After a little practice, it started feeling real good, and for a while those feelings were the *only* feelings I had. I kept doing them because I wanted to know I was alive down there. After I learned to masturbate successfully, I kept doing the exercises because I wanted to increase control in my muscle in order to feel more with intercourse."

STEP 3 SELF-SENSORY EXAMINATION

How: Now you will begin to put to practical use some of the information you learned in Step 1. You know how your genitals look; now it is important to explore how it feels to touch yourself. This preliminary testing of your reactions to touch is essential before starting serious masturbation.

For this exercise you will need some kind of lubricant; you can use saliva, vaginal secretions, or a commercial lubricant or loving oil.

Again, as in Step 1, complete privacy is very important. If at all possible, do this exercise while completely alone in the house. Take the phone off the hook and lock the door. Don't rush through this; take as much time as you need. The exercise usually takes about twenty minutes, but allow yourself plenty of leeway so you don't feel pressured to hurry up and finish before someone interrupts you.

This is *not* an erotic exercise. Referring to Figure 1, facing page 39, rate each part of your genitals as follows: *how* you like it touched: soft, hard, fast, slow, etc.; *how it feels* when you touch it the way you like: good, bad, great, etc. Do this for all the outer genitals indicated on the diagram.

Then draw a circle on your diagram to represent the pubococcygeus muscle in your vagina as a clock. Inserting your finger into your vagina, now test the sensations in your muscle. Find the muscle by putting the tip of your finger about halfway in and squeezing your vagina against your finger. Turn your finger in different directions as you squeeze, and you will feel the closing of a band around your finger. You may have to put your finger in farther or not so far to find this band, which is your pubococcygeus muscle. Rate on the diagram as follows for the sensory test of this muscle:

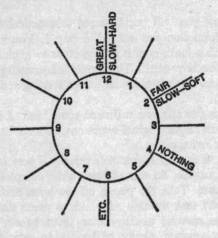

Once you have tested the sensation in a particular part, write your response on the diagram and move on to the next part. When you have tested each part separately, you are finished with the exercise. Do the exercise four or five times a week for as long as six weeks.

You may consider this step completed when you can do it without any anxiety, embarrassment, guilt or shame, and when you feel that you have sufficient information about the subtle differences in sensation between the various parts of both your external genitals and your pubococcygeus muscle to begin masturbation.

If you feel inhibited and anxious about this step, do Step 1 again. It is not unusual to feel uncomfortable doing some of these exercises for the first time, but the more you do them, the less anxiety you will feel. What you are trying to learn is some differences in the sensations in various parts of your genitals. If after six weeks you still don't feel any differences, don't worry. Go on to the next step.

Why: Discovering the sensations in different parts of your genitals before starting masturbation is important, since successful masturbation involves knowing your genitals intimately—what they are, where they are, and how they feel when touched. This is exactly what you need to find out and is the purpose of the self-exam (what and where) and the sensory exam (how it feels).

You must slow down enough to gather this information in a non-stressful situation without seeking arousal or orgasm. Once you know more about your responses, you can then use this information toward those goals.

It is important to complete each step along the way before going on to the next one. Perhaps you feel you have waited too long already for your orgasm, but remember, you still have the rest of your life ahead of you. This is a *learning process,* which means you must take your time. If you were trying to learn to drive a car, you wouldn't just get in and start the engine and expect to be able to drive. You would have to learn the names, locations, and functions of all the instruments, practice operating them, and then start driving in a safe place, eventually moving into areas with more traffic, until you were a competent driver. You learn how to have an orgasm in the same way. The sensory exam is like learning the functions of the instruments.

STEP 4 BEGINNING MASTURBATION

How: Although it may be difficult to arrange, you must be alone in the house when doing this exercise, or at any rate, without anyone around who is old enough to know what you are doing. This is true even for women who think they aren't self-conscious. It is best not to rely on a promise from others in the house that you won't be disturbed. If you are home during the day with young children, do the exercise while they are taking their afternoon naps. In any case, keep your bedroom door closed and *locked*.

If you feel frazzled and tense when you are ready to begin this exercise, take a few minutes to unwind and relax first. If at all possible, try to pick your most energetic time of day to do the exercise.

Using some lubricant and your hand, begin exploring your breasts, your external genitals, and your vagina, slowly and gently. Touch the different parts, individually and simultaneously. Caress both the major and minor labia, and slowly and gradually include the area around the clitoris, and finally the glans, the foreskin, and the shaft of the clitoris itself.

Be as experimental as you can, trying different ways of touching yourself and exploring different sensations. Remember the information you learned from the sensory exam, but don't be restricted by it.

One suggestion for stimulating the breasts is to caress them in a slow, firm movement from the outer area toward the nipple. Then the nipple can be very lightly touched in a "teasing" manner. Alternate between breast and nipple stimulation, gradually increasing the pressure directly on the nipple. Some women enjoy being almost pinched on the nipples, but this is usually after a gradual progression from breast to nipple.

In touching the clitoris, it is important to remember the three parts—the *shaft,* which is the tubelike part below the mons; the *glans,* which is at the bottom of the shaft and looks like a tiny pea; and the *foreskin,* which is the hood or covering of the glans. If the foreskin covers the glans completely, it is necessary to retract it upward to expose the glans to direct touch. These three parts together constitute the clitoris.

The clitoris, like the breasts, can be stimulated in a variety of ways: with the thumb, forefinger, two or three fingers together on one hand, one finger of each hand at the same time, both thumbs, the palm or heel of the hand, the thumbnail or fingernail (lightly), or by using a small cloth to achieve friction. Touch can be in an up-and-down motion, from side to side, or in circular motions that are broad, short, or in between. You can touch from the bottom of the glans upward and over the shaft, and from the shaft down over the glans. You can touch one side of the shaft or the glans or both sides together. (Do not, however, try to stimulate yourself by rubbing against an object such as a pillow. Although many women can become aroused in this manner, it is difficult to add vaginal stimulation to this method of masturbation.) Rhythm can be fast, slow, intermediate, or a combination, and pressure can be light or firm, although in the learning stage it is usually preferable to start with a light touch and gradually increase it as desired.

Try to discover the specific things which increase feeling, and then learn how to decrease feeling gradually by altering the touching, and then increase it again. Some frustration is inevitable here because you are working with such a small area. The distance between the shaft and glans of the clitoris is minute, and moving from one to the other is a very precise operation.

Do not try to have an orgasm at this time. *Your goal is not orgasm, but rather comfort with and exploration of sensations.* Concentrate on allowing yourself to feel all of the sensations to the fullest extent. Do this exercise for twenty minutes, four or five times a week.

You may consider this step completed when you can do it without any anxiety, embarrassment, guilt, or shame, and when you have learned to create some sensation that feels good to you, *even if it doesn't approach arousal;* or after a maximum of six weeks, even if you notice no difference in sensations. In the latter case, which is quite normal, you should merely continue on to the next step; the addition of steps in the following exercises will eventually increase the level of sensations for most women. It is suggested that you not continue on to the next step unless you feel fairly anxiety-free doing this one.

Why: Only if you are alone can you be certain that someone won't be nearby and perhaps listening to your sounds. Nor should you have to listen for the sounds of someone else. You cannot fully relax and concentrate on what you are doing if there is even the slightest possibility of distraction. If you are the least bit concerned about being seen or overheard, part of you will be on guard, and you will not be completely involved in what you are doing. Without that full involvement, you will not feel as much as you would otherwise.

Exceptions to this are very small children who are not consciously aware of what you are doing and won't judge or interpret your behavior. But you must not be distracted by worry about their safety. You must be sure that they are safely in their cribs or beds, that they are sleeping;

you must know how long they will normally sleep, and that they cannot get into any unsafe situation if they do waken suddenly. You must also feel free to make whatever sounds you like without concern over waking them.

A lock on the bedroom door can assure you of being alone even if someone should happen to intrude unexpectedly. Although you would have to stop the exercise, you would not suffer the possible trauma of being "caught in the act."

Relaxation is as important to learning to masturbate as it is to learning any other new activity. If you are tense or fatigued, you simply will not have as much energy to put into it, and your response will be lessened.

The use of a suitable lubricant will reduce friction and increase sensation. And the more sensation you feel, the closer you are to orgasm. However, don't try to have an orgasm at this time, because if you are worrying about having an orgasm, you will not be able to concentrate on your sensations. And if you do not learn to feel sensations first, you will not be able to learn to have an orgasm. To learn to experience orgasm (a concentrated amount of feeling), you must first learn to experience lesser amounts of feeling, and you must also learn to gradually change that amount of feeling from a lesser to a greater amount. Learning to decrease feeling gradually will help you to identify what does not excite you, so that you can better decide what you do like. In addition, if you can create sensation, reduce it, and regain it, this will give you confidence in your ability to recapture sensation. This ability will help prevent you from becoming anxious during lovemaking later.

The time limit of twenty minutes is to prevent you from getting frustrated and discouraged. You are not likely to feel any more *after* twenty minutes than you did *during* the twenty minutes. Your chances of increasing sensation are much greater if you do the exercise in short recurring periods of time when you are rested and relaxed than in long sessions that may become discouraging, tedious, and tiring. Invest your time in the exercises, but do them repeatedly in short sessions.

STEP 5 ADVANCED MASTURBATION

How: Now that you have basic information about your genitals and how to stimulate them, you are ready for more intricate methods of stimulation. You must still do the exercise when you are alone in the house and when you are rested and relaxed.

With your hand, lubricate yourself and begin slowly and gently caressing your outer genitals in the way you liked best in the last step. Begin to focus the touch more directly on the glans area. Develop a rhythm between the shaft, which is less sensitive, and the glans, which is the more sensitive part of the clitoris.

Direct, continuous stimulation of the glans is not enjoyable for most women, so stimulate it enough to arouse you, but not so much that you can't endure it. Stimulate it through the foreskin too, but also try to stimulate it directly. To do this you may need to pull up the foreskin to expose the glans. Work in a regular, recurring rhythm, the way you enjoy it most. Take what you learned about the different physical sensations in the last exercise and focus your concentrations on giving yourself the most pleasure.

Soon, the glans will become more and more sensitive, until it is no longer comfortable to touch it. *Slightly* reduce the amount and frequency of stimulation to the glans, but continue the rhythm you have developed.

It is very important to relax and concentrate solely on your body. Don't worry about trying to feel what you think you ought to feel. Just enjoy the sensations—if you start to worry, you'll lose them.

Eventually, you may feel a flush of warmth and tingling. Enjoy these feelings and continue stimulating yourself with the same rhythm. *Do not stop.* Continue the stimulation until you feel either a flush of warmth and tingling, or a series of automatic vaginal contractions or waves of feeling, and *continue the stimulation until the contractions or waves have stopped.*

Throughout this entire process, you should concentrate on allowing yourself to feel all of the sensations that are there, rather than trying to produce other sensations. Do not try directly to have an orgasm; instead, concentrate on building up as much feeling as possible and allowing yourself to go with, instead of fighting, the feeling.

Do this exercise four or five times a week for twenty minutes each time. Consider this step completed when you can do it without any anxiety, embarrassment, guilt, or shame; and when you can easily masturbate to the pre-orgasmic feeling of warmth, or to an orgasm; or when you have practiced it for six weeks, whichever occurs first. If, after six weeks of following the instructions as outlined, you do not experience at least a pre-orgasmic feeling of warmth, do not be too concerned. This is quite common. The following steps will help increase your chances of success. (Note: If you are easily able to stimulate yourself to orgasm at this point, you may go directly on to Step 11, although it is suggested that you do Steps 6 and 8 first.)

Why: Since the areas which surround the clitoris are somewhat less sensitive than the clitoris itself, you can gradually build up greater sensation from lesser sensation by starting the touch at these points. As you become more and more aroused, you will want to continue the feeling. To do this, you will use direct touch of the clitoris. A light touch at the beginning is important in order to fully "awaken" the nerve endings. A heavy pressure at the start will numb sensation, and once the area becomes numb, sensation cannot be recaptured without waiting perhaps half an hour to an hour.

Many women complain that they cannot tolerate any direct contact of the glans because it is too sensitive, and therefore avoid touching it. This is a mistake. The glans is sensitive for a reason: to enable you to experience enough sensation to be able to reach orgasm. But obviously if the sensation is so strong that you are forced to tighten up all your muscles in protest, you will be unable to have an orgasm. The problem, then, is to find ways to give a little less direct stimulation to a too-sensitive glans, and this is simply a matter of experimenting with technique. If you are like many women who don't feel enough sensation in the glans, simply continue with the rest of the program.

Stimulating the glans through the foreskin will produce a sensation which in intensity is about halfway between shaft stimulation and glans stimulation. It can be used as a stepping stone between the other two sensations.

Touching the shaft produces tolerable levels of sexual stimulation. Although you need the intense direct stimulation of the glans to spur you on to higher levels of sexual sensation, this increase of sexual sensation must be gradual. The stimulation of the shaft keeps you at the level of feeling already obtained without letting you slip back into lesser feeling. (While remembering the similarities between male and female physiology, it is interesting to note that a great many men masturbate by using a combination of glans and shaft stimulation of the penis.)

It is important to keep the stimulation continuous if you are to reach orgasm. The sensation of warmth and tingling which floods the pelvis and sometimes other parts of the body is the point just before actual orgasm. Many women who experience it think this is the complete orgasm and mistakenly discontinue stimulation at this point. If you continue the same stimulation beyond this stage, you will go on to feel the actual orgasm. If you stop the stimulation, even though you already feel the warmth or the contractions, the orgasm may stop. Therefore, you must continue the same stimulation until the entire orgasm is complete.

Orgasm is not something you can will to happen. Even if your technique of stimulation is perfect, orgasm will occur only if you let it. Since you cannot force it, you must forget everything and let your body take over. Orgasm is sensation, and sensation is a body experience, not an intellectual one. It is possible to successfully make orgasm your goal once you know how to stimulate yourself to it with ease, but at the beginning, you must simply allow yourself to fully experience the process of getting there in order to get there at all.

STEP 6 BREATHING AND SOUNDS

How: This exercise is perhaps the most crucial one in the entire masturbation learning program for women who have not yet experienced orgasm, because it is the key to learning to relax sexually.

While alone in the house, practice taking deep breaths and letting them out slowly and deeply with a sighing sound. Imagine that you are in the middle of a pine forest, and that you are as rested and relaxed as you can be. Don't think of anything sexual.

Once you have accomplished this, continue practicing the same breathing and sighing, but think about some sexual act at the same time. Repeat this until you can do it naturally and comfortably.

The next step in this exercise is to escalate this breathing and sighing into a full-blown noise. The sound should be loud and should rattle in the back of the throat as it comes out. Don't push or force the sound out, or choke it back. Just let it flow out easily and fully.

Imagine that the sound is starting way down in your pelvis, traveling all the way up your windpipe, and rattling through the back of your throat on the way out. Practice varying the tone and pitch, so that the sound wavers and goes up and down. Do not screech or scream. Make the sound come out as "ah"; this prevents you from closing off your throat.

Be very careful to breathe as slowly as possible, and to pause a long time between breaths. If you breathe too quickly, you will hyperventilate (which upsets the balance of oxygen and carbon dioxide in your body), causing dizziness, and tingling in the arms, legs, and face. If this happens, breathe at as slow a rate as possible until the symptoms disappear. Then resume the exercise.

When you can do this breathing so that it sounds and feels relaxed and easy to do, continue doing it while imagining that you are doing something sexual. Repeat this until you can do it naturally and comfortably along with your sexual thoughts.

The first four parts of this step can be done at one time or over a period of several days. The fifth and final part is to masturbate as described in Step 5, while at the same time doing the deep breathing and sounds (without a sexual thought) throughout the twenty minutes. Do this for twenty minutes four or five times a week for as long as six weeks.

You may consider this step completed when you can masturbate with breathing and sounds without embarrassment, guilt or shame (taking as long as six weeks to do this); or for a minimum of two weeks if you have no anxieties; or easily to orgasm, whichever occurs first. (Note: If you are easily able to stimulate yourself to orgasm at the completion of this step, you may go directly on to Step 11, although it is suggested that you do Step 8 first.)

Why: The same reasons for being alone in the house still prevail, but here they are even more important, since you are sure to be heard by anyone nearby.

You may find yourself unable to reach high levels of arousal or orgasm even though you are following the technique correctly. Feelings of anxiety which you may not even be aware of can effectively cut off your sensations because you are unconsciously tightening your body or holding your breath, or perhaps you do not feel free to make sounds.

Alexander Lowen, the proponent of bioenergetics, a field of psychotherapy that evolves from the work of Wilhelm Reich, states, "The inability to breathe fully and deeply is also responsible for the failure to achieve full satisfaction in sex. Holding the breath at the approach of climax cuts off the strong sexual sensation. . . . Any restriction on breathing during the sexual act cuts down on the sexual pleasure."[19]

All of these are blocks in awareness; that is, you are not consciously aware of what is occurring in your body. It is important to learn the difference between tension and relaxation. If you can become aware of when your body is tense, you can then make efforts to relax.

It isn't necessary actually to make sounds during a sexual act, but it is necessary to feel free to express sounds if you want to. The only way to have a choice is to feel comfortable with sounds as well as silence. This exercise is to help you feel comfortable with sounds.

The reasoning behind this step is that the easiest thing to do is to breathe and sigh gently. The next easiest thing is to add a sexual thought. It is more difficult to coordinate breathing with a full relaxed sound, and most difficult to do this in association with a sexual thought. Your best chance of accomplishing this fourth step lies in successfully completing the easier steps first.

If you screech, you are not relaxed. One cause of screeching is holding back the sound (tension) or forcing it out unnaturally (tension). What you want to do is something between these two—*let* the sound come out. It is necessary to vary the kind of sounds you make and to experiment until you are sure that the sound you are making is a relaxed one.

When you can do the fourth part of this exercise successfully, it is very unlikely that you will be feeling much anxiety or self-consciousness about "letting go." Even more important, it is almost impossible to use your body to hold back on sensations while you are doing this.

Now you are ready to combine this method of helping yourself relax with the advanced masturbation techniques that you have been practicing. If you do this correctly, the result should be either greatly increased levels of physical sensation, or orgasm.

STEP 7 AUTO-SUGGESTION

How: Using a tape recorder, make the following tape. (Note: If you cannot get a tape recorder, simply read out loud from the book, but a tape is much more effective.) Start the tape and record the following messages:

I masturbate with my hand and I love doing it. Each time I masturbate I feel more and more sensation. Masturbating to orgasm is one of my favorite things to do. It's easy for me to have full, complete orgasms when I masturbate.

When I masturbate I breathe deeply and freely.

I masturbate with my hand and I love doing it. Each time I masturbate I feel more and more sensation. Masturbating to orgasm is one of my favorite things to do. It's easy for me to have full, complete orgasms when I masturbate.

Open-throated sounds come naturally to me when I masturbate.

I masturbate with my hand and I love doing it. Each time I masturbate I feel more and more sensation. Masturbating to orgasm is one of my favorite things to do. It's easy for me to have full, complete orgasms when I masturbate.

When I masturbate it's easy for me to concentrate on feeling all the sensations.

I masturbate with my hand and I love doing it. Each time I masturbate I feel more and more sensation. Masturbating to orgasm is one of my favorite things to do. It's easy for me to have full, complete orgasms when I masturbate.

It's easy for me to totally submit myself to all of my sexual feelings.

I masturbate with my hand and I love doing it. Each time I masturbate I feel more and more sensation. Masturbating to orgasm is one of my favorite things to do. It's easy for me to have full, complete orgasms when I masturbate.

When I masturbate I get carried away by waves of pleasure.

I masturbate with my hand and I love doing it. Each time I masturbate I feel more and more sensation. Masturbating to orgasm is one of my favorite things to do. It's easy for me to have full, complete orgasms when I masturbate.

STOP THE TAPE.

Find a quiet, private place and lie down and relax. Then turn on the tape recorder, shut your eyes, and listen to the tape with as much concentration as you can. Do this twice a day regularly. Meanwhile, at a separate time, continue the advanced masturbation techniques along with the breathing and sounds four or five times a week.

It is not unusual for patients who have not achieved orgasm at this point to begin to feel discouraged. However, there are still other steps in the program which are likely to be helpful for you. In fact, many women never learn to masturbate successfully with their hand but do very well with a vibrator. It's too early at this point to feel discouraged, as success is still quite possible.

Do the auto-suggestion alone twice daily and also continue the advanced masturbation with breathing and sounds. This requires additional time allotments, which admittedly may be very difficult for some women to arrange. Nevertheless, this time commitment is important at this stage of the learning program. You may consider this step completed when you have done it for two weeks, or can easily masturbate to orgasm, whichever occurs first. (Note: If at the end of two weeks you are not having orgasms, go on to the next step. If you reach orgasm, you may go directly on to Step 11, although it is suggested that you do Step 8 first.)

Why: The use of auto-suggestion techniques to communicate directly with the subconscious mind has helped many people. Exactly how auto-suggestion and hypnosis work is still unclear to medical authorities, but they are used extensively in the field of psychiatry.

It is undoubtedly true that if you believe you can do something, you are more likely to be able to do it; conversely, if you are convinced that you can't, you probably won't. The auto-suggestion is intended to bolster your faith in yourself through bypassing as much as possible the conscious mind, which would argue back.

Privacy and relaxation are necessary in order to allow you to concentrate, and the continuation of masturbation is necessary in order to learn to achieve orgasm.

STEP 8 SEXUAL FANTASIES

How: If you are already capable of creating a sexual fantasy in your own mind and using it during a sexual activity, you need not follow the suggestions here about using books and pictures (unless you want to). Simply use your own imagination during the masturbation exercise. However, if you are like a great many other women, either you don't have sexual fantasies, or the fantasies you have are actually much more romantic than sexual, or you may not even know what a fantasy is.

If either of these is true, don't despair. As long as you can read or look at a picture, you can learn to fantasize. Do your fantasizing when you masturbate.

First assemble a small collection of fantasy aids—nude pictures of men and women, either singly or in groups, or pictures of anything else that you find stimulating. Erotic magazines such as *Playgirl, Viva, Playboy* and *Penthouse* are available at most newsstores. Movie magazine photos of your favorite stars are another possibility.

You may also want to take pictures of your favorite man. This can be done with a Polaroid camera. If he is willing, pose him in whatever manner is most provocative to you, which of course will provide a much more real fantasy for you when you use it.

Erotic books are another source of fantasy. Unfortunately, most of the books on the market are intended for a male audience, so a woman has a somewhat difficult time finding one that is likely to arouse her. We provide here a very brief list of books that you may find stimulating. You may use this as a beginner's guide to assembling an erotic collection, or you can disregard it and seek out books on your own. Almost all the books listed are available in any good bookstore, but if you find none of them stimulating, you may want to visit an "adult" bookstore—that is, a store that specializes in erotic merchandise. If so, you may be more comfortable going with a friend instead of alone.

All of the following are available in paperback. One asterisk * stands for classic erotica and two ** for a modern work.

* Anonymous. *The Pearl.* New York: Grove Press, First Evergreen Black Cat Edition, 1968.
* Anonymous. *My Secret Life.* New York: Grove Press, Evergreen Black Cat Edition, 1968.
* Anonymous. *A Man with a Maid.* New York: Grove Press, 1972.
* Cleland, John. *Fanny Hill.* New York: Dell Publishing Company.
** Elbert, Joyce. *Crazy Ladies.* New York: New American Library, 1970.
* Girodias, Maurice, ed. *The Olympia Reader.* New York: Ballantine Books, 1965.
* Harris, Frank. *My Life and Loves.* New York: Grove Press, 1963.
** Lawrence D. H. *Lady Chatterley's Lover.* New York: Bantam Books, 1971.
** Lawrence, D. H. *Women in Love.* New York: Viking Press (also Modern Library).
** Robbins, Harold. *The Adventurers.* New York: Pocket Books, 1972.
** Robbins, Harold. *The Carpetbaggers.* New York: Simon and Schuster, Pocket Books, 1970.
** Yerby, Frank. *The Golden Hawk.* New York: Dell Publishing Company, 1972.
** Yerby, Frank. *The Saracen Blade.* New York: Dell Publishing Company, 1973.

In addition, there are two collections of erotic fantasies: Phyllis and Eberhard Kronhausen's *Erotic Fantasies: A Study of the Sexual Imagination* (New York: Grove Press, First Evergreen Black Cat Edition, 1970);

and Nancy Friday's *My Secret Garden:* Women's Sexual Fantasies (New York: Pocket Books, 1974).

Once you have a few erotica with which to begin this exercise, use them during your masturbation exercises along with breathing and sounds. Try to imagine yourself doing one or more of the sexual acts depicted in the book or picture. Do this for twenty minutes each time, four or five times a week for two weeks. In addition, continue the auto-suggestion twice daily at a separate time.

You need not concentrate exclusively on either books or pictures. They can be used to supplement one another. In other words, you can read a book while bringing in a picture or pictures occasionally—and vice versa. This requires having all your "props" set up ahead of time so that everything is within easy reach.

After you have had repeated successful experiences with erotic materials to arouse yourself during masturbation, and you are able to have an orgasm, you may want to develop your own fantasies, using your own imagination. The most effective way to do this during masturbation is to use a book or picture orgasm. After doing this successfully two or three times, move the point of switchover just a little bit further from the point of orgasm. Continue doing this on a gradual basis until you are able to spend all or most of the time using your own imagination instead of the book or picture.

Erotic movies can be stimulating for many women. A movie can be seen and recalled later before and during masturbation. These movies are available in most large cities and can be found by looking in the local movie guide.

You may consider this step completed when you can masturbate with sexual fantasies (your own, books or pictures) without any anxiety, embarrassment, guilt or shame, taking as long as six weeks to do this; or for a minimum of two weeks if you have no anxieties; or easily to orgasm, whichever occurs first. (Note: If you reach orgasm, go directly to Step 11.)

Why: The previously cited SIECUS report stated that: "Masturbation is usually accompanied by fantasies or daydreams in about three-fourths of the males who masturbate and about half of the females."[20] Kinsey's data seem to indicate that women are less aroused by erotica, but this lack of arousal may be viewed as another example of the difference in social conditioning between men and women in our culture. Actually, Fisher cites two studies in which women were more aroused by erotica than were the males tested.[21]

Helen Kaplan discusses extensively the use of fantasies in helping patients achieve orgasm: "Erotic fantasy during sex is an excellent distractor and is an invaluable tool for overcoming orgastic inhibition. . . . If the inhibited patient consciously focuses her attention on her sexual experience, if she is an 'orgasm watcher,' if she stands apart and judges herself, it is often impossible for her to experience orgasm, even in the face of intense stimulation. Therefore . . . it is very useful to have her focus her attention on an erotic fantasy instead. . . . The trainees in our program refer to this therapeutic maneuver as 'distracting the distractor.' "

Kaplan adds, "However, patients often feel guilty about their sexual fantasies, and they require the therapist's encouragement and reassurance to free them to enjoy their most arousing fantasies during stimulation."[22]

It's easy to understand why so many women feel guilty or don't know how to fantasize if you stop to consider that most women were taught as children to suppress their sexual desires, and hence their sexual thoughts and fantasies. Like any negative conditioning, it is sometimes difficult but very possible to overcome.

If you learned how *not* to fantasize, you can also learn how *to* fantasize. If you learned how to feel guilty about your fantasies, you can also learn how not to feel guilty. The best way to learn is by practice and repetition, and the easiest way to practice is to involve yourself in someone else's fantasies, through a book or a movie. Pictures are a halfway step between someone else's fantasy and your own.

It is common and normal for many men and women to use erotic aids. They are not harmful, in spite of what you may hear from pornography pressure groups. There is no reason to abandon these aids unless you wish to. In most cases, when you have learned to masturbate with the help of books or pictures, you will soon find yourself able to do so without.

Many persons have sexual fantasies. This does not mean that you don't love your partner or that you are dissatisfied with your life in any way. But some women feel frightened or guilty about their fantasies. They may feel that they are perverted in some way. Although sometimes fantasies can indicate that a person is in psychiatric or emotional difficulty, most of the time this is not the case. Since fantasizing is usually a harmless and pleasant experience, it is not necessary to feel guilty about it. It is a safe, private way to experience anything sexually that you desire. The thought of certain sexual acts creates high levels of excitement, and, with more excitement, it becomes more likely that orgasm will occur.

STEP 9 VIBRATOR MASTURBATION

How: The basics of vibrator masturbation are very similar
to the techniques described in Step 5, Advanced Masturbation. If you are already orgasmic with your hand, you
may skip this step and go directly to Step 11.

Using some kind of lubricant and a vibrator, begin
stimulating the outer genitals slowly and gently with the
edge of the vibrating end of the instrument. The vibrator
will be more awkward and clumsy than your own fingers,
but this can be minimized by tipping the vibrator on its
side slightly rather than holding it at a right angle to your
body, so that the smallest part of the vibrating surface
makes contact with the genital area.

Use as light a touch as you can and still feel something.
Gradually begin to focus the touch more directly to the
clitoral area. Develop a rhythm between the shaft, which
is less sensitive, and the glans *through the foreskin,* the
glans being the most sensitive part of the clitoris.

Your goal is to allow enough of the glans stimulation
through the foreskin to be arousing but not so much that
you cannot endure it. The entire process should be one of
a recurring, regular rhythm of these two parts of the clitoris, shaft and foreskin (over glans). It should be done
about six times in succession, with an occasional break to
lift the vibrator off and to replace it directly on the foreskin.

Be sure to add additional lubricant as needed, since vibrator masturbation uses it up much more quickly than
hand masturbation.

As you continue, the glans will become more and more

sensitive until it is no longer comfortable to touch it with the vibrator, even through the foreskin. At this point it is crucial to continue the stimulation in the same manner, except that you may *slightly* reduce the amount and frequency of stimulation to the glans through the foreskin.

As you continue this, you may feel a flush of warmth and tingling. If this occurs you must continue the stimulation in exactly the same manner as before. *Do not stop.* Continue the stimulation until you feel an automatic series of vaginal contractions or waves of feeling. *Continue the stimulation until the contractions or waves have stopped.*

Throughout this entire process, *allow* yourself to feel all of the sensation; don't *try* to produce sensations. *Do not try directly to reach orgasm;* instead, concentrate on building up as much feeling as possible and allowing yourself to go with, rather than resisting, the feeling.

Do this exercise four or five times a week for twenty minutes each time for a period of six weeks. At the end of six weeks, begin adding Steps 6, 7, and 8 as needed in the same manner as with hand masturbation.

You may consider this exercise completed when you can easily masturbate to orgasm with the vibrator. (Note: If you reach orgasm with the vibrator before you have done Steps 6, 7 and 8 with the vibrator, it is suggested that you do Steps 6 and 8 before going on to Step 10.)

Choosing a Vibrator: There are so many different kinds of vibrators on the market that it is impossible to name all of them here. But they fall basically into three categories: battery-powered, electric-powered which fit over your hand, and electric-powered wand type.

For purposes of masturbation we will not consider the type which fits over your hand, since it tends to be awkward and heavy, does not provide adequate stimulation, and tires the hand most easily.

Any battery-powered vibrator is suitable; make sure you are using fresh batteries so you will get enough vibration. This type of vibrator is often phallic-shaped, with a tapered vibrating tip, and is sometimes referred to as a "facial massager." It is carried in many large drugstores as well as by the mail order houses that are listed in some newspapers and magazines. The advantage of this type of vibrator is that the amount of vibration is limited so that it does not tend to create so much dependency on it as do the electric vibrators. Also the cost is small, usually under five dollars, and you can use it without electricity. The disadvantages are that there may not be enough vibration; there is usually no choice of speeds; and batteries must be replaced as they wear down.

There is a great variety of wand-type electric vibrators which are often referred to as "body massagers." The most desirable ones are the small and lightweight ones; they are quiet and provide enough stimulation without being too rough. One that does not heat up quickly is essential; heat on the clitoris can be painful, and pain will prevent orgasm. Electric vibrators have the advantage of giving greater stimulation than battery-powered ones. Since there are no batteries to wear down, the amount of stimulation is always constant. They come complete; there are no parts to replace. With some there is a choice of speeds, to coincide with your needs and responses. Disadvantages are that they are heavier, more clumsy and more expensive than battery vibrators; you are limited to areas with electrical outlets; those with only one speed may be more powerful than you need; and all of them tend to heat up more than battery vibrators do.

Both the battery-type and the electric wand-type vibrators should be used externally on the clitoral area. While we are not aware of any medical studies showing harm from inserting a vibrator in the vagina, to be absolutely safe, it is probably best to avoid insertion.

Why: In her book on sexual therapy, Kaplan refers to the vibrator as: "... the strongest, most intense stimulation known."[23] And the stronger the stimulation, the greater the likelihood of orgasm.

As with hand masturbation, lightness of touch is important; a heavy pressure may initially feel stimulating but will soon greatly reduce sensation, which may not be recovered without a time interval of an hour or more without the vibrator. With the increased intensity of the vibrator, the sensations directly on the glans are usually too stimulating to be pleasant. The foreskin over the glans can serve as a buffer while still allowing as much stimulation as is necessary for arousal. The lifting and replacing of the vibrator on the foreskin provides a different kind of rhythm than is afforded by continual contact and is very arousing.

Again, as you did when you masturbated with your hand, you can incorporate breathing, sounds and sexual fantasies while you are using the vibrator to help you become aroused. Reading a book and using a vibrator at the same time might seem to require three hands, but with patience, practice and a sense of humor, you'll be able to manage. Use the auto-suggestion twice a day too, and incorporate these steps into your sessions at the same rate as you did for manual masturbation.

If after three weeks you don't have an orgasm with the vibrator, don't despair. It doesn't mean that you won't be able to learn how. Perhaps you didn't follow the instructions correctly. Perhaps you didn't spend the required time on the exercise. If you feel you rushed through them, go back and start again. It is possible you don't really care whether you are having orgasms or not, but are trying to do so in order to satisfy your partner. Remember, you can be warm, loving, sexy and responsive without having orgasms. You can also be a perfectly satisfactory sex partner. What counts is whether *you* are satisfied with yourself and with sex.

It is also possible that you have some deep-seated traumatic feelings to overcome. In this case you should seek psychiatric help, not because you are "abnormal," but so that you can be freed to be the sexual person you really are.

STEP 10 TAPERING OFF THE VIBRATOR

How: Tapering yourself off vibrator masturbation and switching to hand masturbation is basically the same as making the transition from erotic books to your own fantasies. But do this only if you are able to masturbate to orgasm easily several times with the vibrator. If you do not wish to abandon the vibrator for hand masturbation, skip this step and go on to the next one.

Masturbate with the vibrator in your usual manner. As your orgasm begins, remove the vibrator with one hand, and with the other hand continue to stimulate yourself, duplicating as closely as you can the kind of stroking you were doing with the vibrator. If you lose the orgasm completely, use the vibrator again, and then switch to your fingers as the orgasm begins. Try this up to three times in one masturbating session, and if you are unable to complete your orgasm with your hand, finish up with the vibrator. Continue this each time you masturbate until you can easily finish your orgasm with your hand instead of the vibrator.

When you have mastered the above, move the moment

of bringing in your hand further and further away from the point of orgasm. This should be done very gradually over as much time as it takes. Eventually you will reach a point where you will use the vibrator only to begin stimulation, or where you will not need it at all.

Masturbate four or five times a week during this tapering-off process. The normal period of time for a complete switch from vibrator to hand masturbation is several weeks. This step is completed when you can easily masturbate to orgasm with your hand.

Why: There is nothing wrong, second-rate, or abnormal about masturbating with a vibrator. Therefore, there is no necessity to taper yourself off it unless you want to. LoPiccolo reports: "In one case, the client is orgasmic one hundred percent of the time, provided her husband stimulates her clitoris with the vibrator during intercourse. We felt somewhat dissatisfied with this outcome, and designed a stimulus generalization program to gradually fade out the electric vibrator for this woman. She quite correctly resisted this. ... She also pointed out, 'There is nothing intrinsically evil about electricity,' and was thus able to convince us to stay out of her now very satisfying sex life."[24]

If you find masturbating with a vibrator completely satisfactory, don't bother to change. You are perfectly normal, and so is your method of masturbating. There is no need to masturbate with your hand simply because other women might wish to. You should be concerned with satisfying your own sexual desires, not those of others.

However, a great many of the female patients seen at the clinic have reported that they are dissatisfied at being "hooked" on the vibrator—that is, unable to alter the pattern of their sexual response. For them, being "hooked" creates a problem because they want to be able to have an orgasm with a partner rather than just by themselves. Once they develop a pattern of response to the intense stimulation of the vibrator, often a partner's hand simply does not provide enough stimulation to promote orgasm. This sometimes leaves the woman in a very frustrating situation. Masturbation is certainly better than not having an orgasm at all, but if this is the only way a woman can have orgasms, it can create a tremendous amount of anger, sadness and poor communication between the woman and her partner, sometimes precipitating the end of the relationship. A man often feels that there is something wrong with him when his partner can respond to a vibrator but not to him. Or he may feel that there is something wrong with her, and the woman frequently agrees with him. (However, some couples successfully integrate the use of the vibrator in love play and intercourse and are completely satisfied with this technique.)

It is because of these problems that this program emphasizes manual masturbation as a first step even though vibrator masturbation may seem to be quicker and easier to learn. However, it is important to state that many women are perfectly capable of being orgasmic with the vibrator and also are able to have an orgasm with manual or oral stimulation as well as intercourse. In fact, often it is easier to learn to have the first few orgasms with a vibrator, and then, once a woman knows just what an orgasm feels like, to learn how to masturbate with her hand.

You may have other reasons for wanting to stop using the vibrator. It is often inconvenient to take it with you whenever you want to masturbate and difficult and impractical to take it to places where you may want to use it.

By gradually changing the moment of introducing your hand in the tapering-off process, you can be successful because you are only trying to change a very small part of your technique at a time. Small changes are more similar to the original technique than large changes, and are more likely to allow you to continue having your usual sexual response.

STEP 11
ADDING VAGINAL PUBOCOCCYGEAL STIMULATION

How: This step is necessary for those women who wish to be orgasmic with intercourse. For those already orgasmic during intercourse, practicing this step will greatly increase vaginal sensation and allow orgasm to be reached more easily. The addition of pubococcygeal stimulation to your present masturbation technique must be gradual. You will need something with which to stimulate your vaginal muscle; you may simply use a finger, or you can use any safe penis substitute, such as a "dildo" (an artificial penis) of moderately small proportions. If you find it awkward to use your finger and difficult to purchase a "dildo," a substitute available to any woman is a new, clean table candle.

Masturbate in your usual manner, with the vaginal stimulator resting in the vagina. Continue masturbating until you reach orgasm. The next time you masturbate, leave the vaginal stimulator in the vagina as you did before, but begin moving it gently as you are having your orgasm. If this is too distracting to allow orgasm, stop the movement and rearouse yourself. As you begin your orgasm, start gentle movement of the stimulator again. Try this up to three times in one masturbating session, and if you are unable to complete your orgasm with movement of the vaginal stimulator, finish up with the stimulator resting in the vagina.

When you can easily accomplish the above, move the moment of adding the pubococcygeal stimulation further and further away from the point of orgasm, and gradually increase the vigor of the movement to stimulate actual intercourse. This should be done very gradually over as much time as it takes. In addition, you may wish to contract your pubococcygeal muscle during masturbation as you are able to tolerate additional pubococcygeal sensation. This squeezing of the muscle creates an increase in the amount of feeling which is usually a distraction until a woman learns to enjoy the sensation as part of the arousal process.

Masturbate four or five times a week for twenty minutes or to orgasm, whichever comes first. Eventually you will reach a point where the vaginal stimulation ceases to be a distraction and becomes a part of the arousal process. (This may take weeks, or even months, to occur, depending on the frequency of masturbation.) You may consider the exercise completed when this happens, but *you should continue to masturbate in this manner most of the time from now on.*

Why: The reason for learning to have your first orgasms with clitoral stimulation alone is that this is the easiest and least complex way of learning. However, during intercourse the clitoris receives only indirect stimulation, from traction on the clitoral foreskin, and sometimes more directly from pubic bone contact; therefore, adequate vaginal stimulation is an integral part of the arousal process. This is difficult to accomplish if a woman has never associated vaginal stimulation with her sexual feelings.

The easiest and least stressful way to associate vaginal stimulation with sexual response is to practice during masturbation, until the vaginal stimulation itself becomes part of the arousal which leads to orgasm. At this point, your chances of experiencing orgasm from this same type of vaginal stimulation, intercourse, are very good even without simultaneous direct clitoral stimulation.

In order to maintain this association between clitoral and vaginal stimulation, it is recommended that most of the time you continue to masturbate stimulating both areas. This will pose no difficulty, since at this point the vaginal stimulation should be as important to arousal as clitorial stimulation.

As with some aspects of this program, small changes are more similar to the original successful technique than large changes and are more likely to allow you to continue to have your usual sexual response. The method of gradually adding more and more movement of the vaginal stimulator is successful because you are only trying to change a small part of your technique at a time.

Note: If you have been unsuccessful with this part of the program, don't be discouraged. It is inherent in any "do it yourself" instructions that they are easy for some and difficult for others. If you have been unsuccessful, it may still be helpful for you to go on to the next chapter. Although in general it is important to follow the recommended sequence of steps, people are not machines, and occasionally in clinical practice a woman succeeds in having her first orgasm with a partner instead of alone.

It happens frequently that a woman experiencing her first orgasm does not recognize that she has had an orgasm. Many women feel vaginal contractions but no sensation of warmth; some experience waves of sensation but no vaginal contractions; still others experience something new and different but can't define it clearly. Learning to identify, experience and observe orgasm often takes time and patience. In some women it takes months to become fully orgasmic. Don't be unduly hard on yourself. If you were learning to play tennis, you wouldn't put yourself down for having to start against the backboard, or for not being as good as Billie Jean King. Don't compare yourself with others—just compare yourself with yourself, and give yourself some credit for what you have done, and for having had the courage to try. And give yourself some time.

Finally, if you feel you have tried everything and are discouraged and disillusioned, you should seek psychiatric help. With appropriate help, any woman who does not have a physical disorder should be able to achieve orgasm.

For those who have succeeded with this chapter, the following chapter deals with the next learning level: being able to enjoy full sexual satisfaction with a partner.

SUMMARY OF THE ELEVEN-STEP PROGRAM FOR ACHIEVING SELF-STIMULATED ORGASM

Step One

1. Arrange for privacy.
2. Using a hand mirror, carefully examine your genitals and breasts for detail and compare yourself to the illustration facing page 39.
3. Spend at least ten minutes each time you do the exercise.
4. Repeat four or five times a week.

Step Two

1. While standing, sitting, or lying down, squeeze the

vagina (pubococcygeus muscle) together without using the abdomen.

2. Use a six-second count for maximum results:

   1: a slow, steady contraction of the vagina;

   2: hold steady;

   3: continue to hold steady;

   4: continue to hold steady:

   5: extra squeeze while using your abdominal muscles;

   6: relax the muscle fully.

3. Repeat for five minutes three times a day or a total of fifteen minutes daily.

Step Three

1. Referring to Figure 1, facing page 39, rate each part of the external genitals as to how you like it touched.

2. Rate each part of the external genitals as to how it feels when you touch it.

3. Rate each part of the pubococcygeus muscle in the vagina as to how you like it touched.

4. Rate each part of the pubococcygeus muscle in the vagina as to how it feels when you touch it.

5. Do the exercise four or five times a week.

Step Four

1. Using lubricant, slowly and gently explore your breasts and outer genitals as well as the vagina, starting with the labia and areas around the clitoris, and then including the glans, foreskin, and shaft of the clitoris.

2. Be as experimental as you can in trying different kinds of touch and experiencing different sensations.

3. The goal is *not* orgasm, but rather gradually increasing levels of sensation and arousal.

4. Do this for twenty-minute periods, four or five times a week while alone in the house.

Step Five

1. Slowly and gently begin caressing your outer genitals, using lubricant.

2. As you begin to stimulate the clitoris, develop a rhythm between the shaft and the glans, giving yourself always just enough glans stimulation to create increasing levels of sexual feeling.

3. When the glans becomes too sensitive, reduce the amount and frequency of glans stimulation *slightly, but continue to use the same technique and continue stimulating yourself.*

4. If you feel a flush of warmth and tingling, or automatic vaginal contractions or waves of feeling, *continue the stimulation in exactly the same manner until your orgasm is completed.*

5. Don't try specifically to have an orgasm; instead, allow yourself to fully feel all the sensations in the *process* of reaching orgasm.

6. Do this while alone in the house for twenty minutes four or five times a week.

Step Six

1. Practice deep breathing along with sighing sounds.

2. Add a sexual thought to the breathing and sighing sounds.

3. Continue the breathing, but change the sighing into a loose, free, easy, naturally flowing loud "ah" sound that rattles out of the throat.

4. Add to this a sexual thought.

5. Do this (without a sexual thought) during the advanced masturbation techniques that you have been prac-

ticing, for twenty minutes a day, four or five times a week.

Step Seven

1. Make a tape recording of the auto-suggestion wording under "How."

2. Listen to it twice a day in privacy (not during your masturbation exercises).

3. At a separate time, continue advanced masturbation four or five times a week with breathing and sounds.

Step Eight

1. Masturbate using advanced masturbation techniques, breathing, and sounds, and at the same time read an erotic book that appeals to you, or look at erotic pictures which arouse you while imagining that you are doing something sexual with the person(s).

2. Continue auto-suggestion twice daily at a separate time.

3. Do this for twenty minutes a day, four or five times a week.

Step Nine

1. Using lubricant, slowly and lightly begin stimulating the outer genitals with the edge of the vibrating end of a vibrator.

2. As you begin to stimulate the clitoris, develop a rhythm between the shaft and the foreskin over the glans, giving yourself always just enough glans stimulation to create increasingly higher levels of sexual feeling.

3. When the glans becomes too sensitive, reduce the amount and frequency of glans stimulation *slightly*, but

continue to use the same technique and continue stimulating yourself.

4. Add breathing and sounds, sexual fantasies, and auto-suggestion twice a day at a separate time, in the same manner as you did with hand masturbation.

5. If you feel a flush of warmth and tingling, or automatic vaginal contractions or waves of feeling, *continue the stimulation in exactly the same manner until your orgasm is completed.*

6. Don't try specifically to have an orgasm; instead allow yourself to fully feel all the sensations in the *process* of reaching orgasm.

7. Do this while alone in the house for twenty minutes four or five times a week.

Step Ten

1. Masturbate with the vibrator in your usual way.

2. As your orgasm begins, remove the vibrator with one hand and with the other hand continue to give yourself stimulation, duplicating the kind of stroking that you were doing with the vibrator as closely as you can.

3. Continue this each time you masturbate until you can easily finish your orgasm with your hand.

4. From then on each time you masturbate, gradually move the moment of bringing in your hand further and further away from the point of orgasm.

5. Masturbate four or five times a week for twenty minutes at a time.

Step Eleven

1. Masturbate to orgasm in your usual manner with the addition of a vaginal stimulator resting quietly in your vagina.

2. The next time you masturbate, use the same

method, but as your orgasm begins, *gently* move the vaginal stimulator, and continue this for the duration of the orgasm.

3. Continue this each time you masturbate until you can easily finish your orgasm while experiencing very gentle vaginal stimulation.

4. From then on, each time you masturbate, gradually move the moment of bringing the vaginal stimulation further and further away from the point of orgasm, and gradually increase the vigor of the movement to simulate actual intercourse.

5. Masturbate four or five times a week for twenty minutes at a time.

CHAPTER 3

A Ten-Step Program for Achieving
Orgasm with Intercourse

The inability to achieve climax during intercourse is a devastating problem for many women. Countless numbers of these women fake orgasm rather than say no to the inevitable question, "Did you come?"

This chapter sets out a step-by-step program for achieving orgasm with intercourse. Indeed, this text would be incomplete if it provided a learning program for only the "solo" orgasm. For although masturbation is a uniquely gratifying experience, so is intercourse. Sexual satisfaction during lovemaking with a partner is an important part of a woman's full sexual experience. Sex as a shared experience is one of life's greatest pleasures.

Those who state that sex without love is equal to sex with love have never experienced sex with love. Couples who love each other and enjoy a measure of honesty and intimacy have a far greater chance of having really satisfying sexual experiences. Love makes the sex better, and sex makes the love better. But it is possible for sex without love to be good, and it is possible for a woman to achieve sexual satisfaction and orgasm without love. Men have done this for centuries, and in spite or poetic notions to the contrary, women are capable of the same. What is important is that a woman be able to have an orgasm when and where *she* wants to. And if and when a woman does become involved in a love relationship, that relationship will be all the more enhanced by her ability to be sexually responsive, just as it is for men.

A woman must have her orgasm for herself. This program is set up in such a fashion that the primary responsibility for the woman's orgasm remains with her. You are not trying to have an orgasm with your partner to please *him* but to please yourself. If you try to produce an orgasm for your partner, you will be under tremendous pressure to perform; you will become a spectator at your own performance, and most likely you will be unable to succeed. Even during intercourse, your orgasm is yours, and nobody else can have it for you. You must attain and experience it for yourself.

Some women automatically become orgasmic with intercourse after successfully completing the masturbation program outlined in the previous chapter. If you are one of these women, it is not necessary to follow the steps in this chapter, although you and your partner may wish to do them together for your mutual enjoyment. In addition, Steps 7 and 8, which can be done without any special cooperation from your partner during intercourse, are important for any woman to do. They will increase sensation for you during intercourse, which is beneficial even if you are already orgasmic with intercourse.

If you are already able to achieve orgasm with masturbation and are beginning this chapter, *you should first complete Step 11 of the previous chapter.*

Because of the different ways men and women are sexually conditioned in this society, men are generally quicker to reach sexual excitement. For this reason, non-genital touching first, and later genital stimulation before actual intercourse, helps a woman "warm up." The more excited you are before penetration, the greater the likelihood of an orgasm during intercourse. Therefore, in all of the steps which include intercourse, a period of foreplay is suggested first. You should direct and participate actively in this pre-coital touching. Steps 1 and 2 will instruct you how to do this. Once you learn to have an orgasm with intercourse, this pre-coital touching will not always be necessary, but it will probably always help you to reach orgasm and will be very enjoyable for both partners.

Do not predetermine the period of time it will take you to reach your ultimate goal of orgasm. Each exercise has an end point, and that should be your only objective. Ideally, each step should be done separately, one at a time and in the proper sequence. This program, which has been used successfully in clinical practice with hundreds of female patients and is built on solid theoretical concepts, approaches the problem one step at a time; the goal is achieved by successive gains, each built upon the last. However, if you do not have a steady partner, you may vary the sequence according to your situation.

Although all of the steps in this chapter are a logical sequence to those of the previous chapter, there will still be some women who will not be able to achieve orgasm with intercourse even if they have followed the instructions carefully. Poor tone of the pubococcygeus muscle will account for some of these failures, even in cases where the actual control and strength of the muscle are good. (See Part 3, Chapter 1.) Another element which is often important in determining whether or not a woman will be orgasmic with her partner is the quality of the relationship. LoPiccolo, in analyzing his treatment failures with situational orgasmic dysfunction (women who are able to reach orgasm with masturbation but not with intercourse), found the quality of the relationship and the ability to resolve conflict the crucial factors in determining success or failure.[1] An intimate, loving relationship is not always necessary in order for a woman to have an orgasm with her partner, but a poor relationship can prevent a woman from trusting her partner enough to allow herself to have one with him. A woman may mistrust men in general, because of early or later experiences; she may be fearful that the relationship isn't going to last; she may believe that the man is being or has been unfaithful to her; or he may be totally or partially withdrawn from her. A lot of hurt and anger between the couple or a lack of real communication can negatively affect the woman trying to have an orgasm with intercourse. Where this is true, the physical practices outlined in this chapter should be followed, but in addition the relationship itself has to be improved in order for orgasm to occur. This requires, in almost every instance, psychotherapy aimed at helping both persons to learn how to listen to each other; to acknowledge what they have heard; to share their feelings honestly without passing judgment on each other; to be sensitive to each other's feelings; and to share their love in such a way that each can give and receive it. Couples who do not harbor negative feelings toward each other can usually learn this fairly easily, but those who have accumulated hurts and resentments over the years have a longer process to go through before they can begin to listen, let alone talk to each other. Once the negative feelings have been dealt with and the couple have established a measure of honesty and intimacy, orgasm is usually easily learned.

Although the above factors apply more to the long-term marital or committed relationship than to the casual, non-committed one, we have discovered in our clinical experience that women can learn to achieve orgasm during intercourse without being in a committed relationship. However, for this program to be successful, the casual partner should be a person you can trust. He should be someone with whom you can honestly share your feelings, since you will need to discuss with him your inability to achieve orgasm. And he must care enough to be a willing participant in the program. A man who meets these qualifications is usually someone you have known for more than a brief time. In sum, your partner should be someone with whom you feel comfortable and relaxed, and whom you feel you can trust, regardless of the degree of commitment in the relationship.

In order to successfully complete the steps in this chapter, you will need the cooperation of your partner. He should be receptive to your level of sexual development and responsiveness, empathetic without being overly concerned, emotionally supportive, encouraging, loving and, above all, willing to let you take responsibility for your own progress. Any notions he may have about "giving" you your orgasms will sabotage your chances of success. Any machismo must be left outside the bedroom door.

In order for you to have ample opportunity to experience sensation during intercourse, which is of course a prelude to orgasm, intercourse must last a certain period of time. Anywhere from five to ten minutes will probably be ample time to experience sensations. If your partner is unable to maintain an erection for this length of time, it could hamper your progress. If he has difficulty with premature ejaculation or maintaining an erection, it would be wise for him to seek help from a sexual therapist. These problems are fairly easily treated (especially premature ejaculation) and are frequently found in association with a woman's inability to climax during intercourse. Periods of intercourse lasting twenty minutes or more should be discouraged, as they do not help the woman, and they may foster male sexual difficulties.

Achieving an orgasm with a partner is somewhat more complex than achieving an orgasm alone. You will always have some concern for your partner, which can easily be escalated into concern about what he thinks about your progress or lack of it. While sensitivity to your partner and caring are important to any good relationship, over-sensitivity, or caring more about how *he* thinks you are doing than what *you* think, can be dangerous.

Before you begin any of these steps with your partner, have a long talk with him and let him know what you expect of him and of yourself. Find out to what extent he is willing to cooperate with you, and keep the channels of communication open throughout the time that you do the exercises. If, in the process of doing these steps, your feelings change, or his do, rediscuss it. It is a good idea to set aside at least a few minutes to really share your feelings with each other at the conclusion of each exercise each time you do it, so each of you will know what the other's reactions are. This will prevent any unpleasant surprises for either of you.

If you or your partner don't want to do certain of the steps, skip those steps and go through the rest in sequence. You can do Steps 7, 8, 9 and 10 without any special cooperation from your partner, except that they do require a partner in order to have intercourse.

If you follow the instructions and find that you are not successful, it does not mean that you will never be. After making certain that the condition of your pubococcygeus muscle is good, and after ruling out any other physical abnormalities, you should consider seeking the help of a qualified sex therapist or psychotherapist. Often there are unconscious blocks preventing a woman from experiencing her full sexual potential, and these can be uncovered and dealt with with the help of a therapist.

There is a summary of steps after Step 10 for your ease in following the program, but it should be used only after reading all of the steps in the text completely.

STEP 1 COMMUNICATION EXERCISE

How: This is a sensuous exercise, not a sexual one, for you and your partner to do together. Although this is best done with a steady partner, it can be done with a non-steady partner as well. If you do not wish to do this together, skip this step and go on to the next one.

The exercise takes about three hours, so the best times are after a light breakfast in bed or after a light supper in the evening. You must be sure that you won't be interrupted; otherwise the feeling of intimacy you are building up may be lost. Take the phone off the hook, unplug it or smother it with pillows and turn it down low. Lock the front door and the bedroom door if there are others living in the house—and make sure that the others are occupied.

Begin by taking a bath together. Use some sweet-scented soap that you both like, and perhaps some bath oil or bubble bath. Don't try to arouse your partner; you should both concentrate on relaxing. Using soap and water, slowly and gently caress your partner's body, trying to feel as much as you can while you do the washing. Wash your partner all over, including the genital area. Wash each other simultaneously if you like. Keep the conversation limited to exchanging feelings about what you are doing.

If the bathtub is too small, one of you might sit on a stack of pillows next to the tub and wash the other without having to strain as you lean over. If you don't have a bathtub, shower together. A bath is a slower and more relaxing process, though.

After your bath, dry the other person all over and move into another room for the rest of the exercise.

Without clothes, sit in a comfortable position facing each other. Take your partner's hands in your own and, starting at the top of your head, show him and tell him how you like to be touched in one small place only (such as scalp, or hair). He should tell you that he understands what you are saying, and at the same time show you by doing to you, without your help, what you have just shown him. If he is doing it the way you like, tell him so, and then switch roles. If he is not doing it the way you like, re-explain it to him and show him again until he understands and can do it alone while repeating your instructions. Continue alternating back and forth until all non-genital areas of both of your bodies are explored. Then do the same for the breasts and genital areas.

Divide your body into as small areas as you can (for instance, scalp, temples, hair, forehead, nape of neck, etc.). Although this does require a lot of time, it is very rewarding even for those couples who have excellent sexual communication. The important point is *not* that your partner find out what you like or how you like it; you are each to take active responsibility in discovering what you like, even for those areas where you may not have any idea, such as the elbow, and then communicate that information to your partner in such a way that he/she can understand it.

Spend as much time as you need, immediately upon finishing, to share with each other all of your feelings about the exercise. Start with the negative feelings first.

Try to say what you *would have liked*, not what you didn't like, and be sensitive to your partner while doing this. Finish up with what you did like.

This exercise is completed when you both feel that you have sufficient information about yourself and your partner to begin using it in lovemaking. Some couples will feel ready for this after doing the exercise only once, while others may wish to repeat it once or several times.

Why: By washing each other all over at the beginning of the exercise, you ensure your own and your partner's cleanliness; you then feel comfortable enough to be physically intimate without worrying about offending or being offended. For those who are attracted by the sexual scent of their partner, which is especially prevalent in the genital area, less soap, or just water, can be used in these areas. Water temperature, of course, must be comfortable for both persons in order for the exercise to be enjoyable. Conversation during the bath is limited to exchanging feelings about what you are doing, to allow for a feeling of closeness and intimacy to be built up, which would be destroyed by talking about other matters.

The objective of the exercise is for each of you to increase your ability to communicate directly and concisely your sexual/sensual likes and dislikes; and to take active responsibility in discovering what you like. This is a very different concept from finding ways to arouse your partner—instead, you are finding ways to arouse yourself, so your partner isn't pressured and anxious trying to figure it out, which becomes very difficult indeed when even *you* don't know.

As we said earlier, women are encouraged to dress, act, and relate seductively, but are given very strict rules for when and where they can actually do anything sexual. Her lack of practice and experience shows in the way a woman relates sexually with her partner. She often does not know what to do to him, or what to have him do to her. In other words, being ignorant of how her lover can give pleasure to her, both genitally and non-genitally, she is ignorant of how to give pleasure to herself. Instead, she depends on him to do this for her, thus perpetuating her lack of knowledge. And the man, although he is usually aware of what he likes, spends his time trying to figure out what she likes instead of enjoying his own feelings. As Masters and Johnson have said:

"The most unfortunate misconception our culture has assigned to sexual functioning is the assumption by both men and women that men by divine guidance and infallible instinct are able to discern exactly what a woman wants sexually and when she wants it. Probably this fallacy has interfered with natural sexual interaction as much as any other single factor."[2]

Most people have one goal in lovemaking—that both partners be sexually satisfied. Most people are taught to accomplish this by taking responsibility for each other's enjoyment and "working each other up." However, just as you are unable to taste and enjoy your partner's meal for him, you are incapable of feeling your partner's sexual response; they are trapped within his body, as yours are trapped within yours. Since you are the only one who can experience your sensations or know when you are feeling them, it only makes good sense to take the responsibility necessary to achieve these sensations. This does not mean that you should never do anything sexually for your partner. If you wish to do something for him, let him know clearly and directly, and do whatever you both agree to. But feel free to stop when you no longer wish to continue, knowing that you don't *have* to continue, because he can satisfy himself. (The same applies in the reverse situation.)

If you follow this line of reasoning to its conclusion, you will understand that if both accept responsibility for satisfying themselves, the goal of two satisfied partners is achieved without the "performance" anxiety that so greatly interferes with sexual sensation.

Once you know what you like, you can use the information yourself. But if you wish to have your partner use the information, you must be able to tell him. This exercise allows you to practice doing that. Since a great many people are raised with the idea that selfishness is a sin, it becomes difficult to communicate in areas where you are seeking some kind of pleasure. But it is important to be able to do so when relating sexually to someone else. At the clinic this exercise is usually one of the most popular and eye-opening steps for couples seen in treatment.

In order to get the most out of sex, you must begin to look at your sex life in terms of what you can do for yourself—not what your partner is doing wrong.

STEP 2 PLEASURING

How: This exercise is for you and your partner to do together. If you or your partner don't want to do this together, skip this step and go on to the next one.

You are now going to take the information you gained from the last exercise about what you like and use it to pleasure yourself. If you have a steady partner, you will also be using the information about what he likes. Pleasuring, as used by sexual therapists, is essentially the same thing as foreplay, except that it does not precede anything else, and it is intended to feel good to both partners, not just the woman. In this exercise don't try to arouse your partner. Enjoy the exercise itself.

Don't feel that you must remember everything you did and discussed from the previous step. Just use the information that you do remember, and if you wish to refresh your memory, repeat the previous step, or part of it, anytime you care to.

These are to be caresses, not massages. The purpose of these exercises is to pleasure yourself, not your partner. As long as your partner is feeling either neutral or positive about receiving, and you are in the mood, go ahead. If your partner actually feels negative about being touched, postpone the exercise to another time.

Since you are doing this for yourself, you needn't be concerned about your partner's reaction. If he actually *dislikes* what you are doing, he should speak up and tell you. If you don't hear from him, don't worry about it. One way you can help yourself touch without concern for his reaction is to do the exercise without words and with both of you keeping your eyes closed. If you can't see him, you can't tell from his face how he might be feeling. After the exercise, plan on sharing your feelings with each other in the same manner as you did previously.

Part 1—Facial Caress:

1. Decide who will be the "giver" and who will be the "receiver." It will be the giver's role to give for himself or herself and the receiver's role to relax and enjoy as much as he or she can.

2. Spend ample time in getting yourselves into positions that will be comfortable for each of you. A possible position is with the giver sitting up in bed, leaning on pillows against the headboard, the receiver lying on his back with his head between the giver's legs. This allows

the giver full access to the other's face without back strain.

3. Make sure that the room is warm enough: as the receiver relaxes, the metabolism will slow down, causing him to feel chilly.

4. Use some lubricant—oil or lotion—if you wish to reduce friction and facilitate the movement of skin sliding over skin. Pour a small amount in your palm and rub your hands together to warm it before applying it to your partner's face. (You may substitute baby powder on other parts of the body; but be careful to avoid breathing it into your lungs, as this can be dangerous.)

5. Start by cupping your hands around his chin, and slowly, while counting silently to twenty, bring your hands on either side of his face up to the forehead.

6. Imagine that his face is made of velvet. You want to feel all of it without applying any pressure. Use the full hand, your fingers, and especially palms, to caress his face. Try to make as much contact as you can.

7. Make sure that your thumbs follow the rest of the hand. If they stick up in the air, it is a sign of tension on your part. Take a deep breath and try to relax, forcing your thumbs down with the fingers.

8. Close your eyes. Imagine that you have lost the power of sight. Try to find out what he looks like with your hands. Concentrate on the feeling going into your hands and arms without seeing. Do this for at least five minutes.

9. Give yourself permission fully to explore his face. Let your fingers and hands travel all over. Find the ears, the mouth. Go inside the lips with a finger. Touch the gums and the insides of the cheeks. Feel the wetness.

10. Have him take his hands and place them on top of yours. Allow your hands to go limp, and let him direct them to the places he wants touched. He can indicate

what kind of pressure he likes, firm or light. When he has communicated his message, he can take his hands away.

11. Use the information gained to *pleasure yourself*. You are under no pressure or obligation to continue touching him in the same way, but if it pleases you to do so, go ahead.

12. Switch roles and repeat, preferably on a different day.

13. Do *not* go on to additional sexual contact at this time, as the point of the exercise is to help you learn to re-focus your goal away from orgasm *per se* to experiencing various sensations.

Part 2—Body Caress Without Genitals:

Again, as with the facial caress, make certain that you are both in comfortable positions before you start. Use the same slow touching as described above with the facial caress, and, again, lubricant if you wish. Although you should feel free to touch his entire body, don't feel pressured to do so. Take a lot of time on each part; get to know your lover's body inch by inch. Imagine that you are on an exploring trip. Later, as a variation, you can use your face, breasts, lips, feet, etc., to caress with instead of your hands. Do *not* go on to additional sexual contact at this time.

Switch roles and repeat, preferably on a different day.

Part 3—Body Caress with Genitals:

This is to be given in the same manner as the body caress without genitals, except that after a period of time spent on touching just the non-genital areas, you should also touch the breasts and genitals. The exercise should last about twenty minutes. Do *not* go on to additional sexual contact at this time.

You may consider this step completed when you can give each other these caresses in such a way as to give pleasure to yourselves without trying to satisfy your partner. Some couples will feel ready to go on after doing each part only once, while others may wish to repeat that part once or several times.

Why: A massage is nice to receive, but often strenuous to give, and the giver gets very little out of it physically for himself. A caress, however, can be enjoyable to give as well as to receive, since you can enjoy the sensations of touching your partner with your own body at the same time as you are giving him pleasure. A caress can be defined as slowly and lightly touching the other person, without actually stimulating the muscles underneath the skin. Although the touch is light, it needn't tickle; it can be a solid, firm-handed kind of touch without massaging the muscles.

The objective of this exercise is for each of you to continue taking active responsibility in discovering what you like; to find ways in which to satisfy yourself physically while at the same time making contact with your partner, thus relieving your partner of the burden of having to do it; to allow your partner to arouse him/herself from the contact against your body; and to begin to have some real, open, honest communication about your likes and dislikes physically and sexually.

It is important to take turns being the *giver* and the *receiver*. The giver's responsibility is to give for herself, in such a way as to please herself. It is toward this goal that she should exert herself. It is the receiver's responsibility to let the giver know if he is feeling negative about what is happening. This is the easiest way for the giver to find out, and relieves her of having to worry about it needlessly. It is quite possible for the receiver not to be feeling much of anything during the exercise, that is, not particularly positive or particularly negative. This is a perfectly valid "response" (or lack of response). It is not necessary for the receiver to be feeling positive about receiving in order to continue the exercise, although he should not be feeling negative.

Most women's sexual responses are somewhat in "slow motion" compared to their partner's, due to the differences in the way they were brought up. So while a man may be very ready for intercourse, a woman may be just getting interested. Unless she has the opportunity to relax, her anxieties can easily prevent her from experiencing any strong sexual sensations. A period of mutual pleasuring preceding penetration can provide this opportunity, but only if the woman (or the man) feels completely free to end the contact at any point without feeling obligated to continue on to full intercourse.

In addition, a woman seeking orgasm, which is something she must give to and experience herself, must practice seeking less anxiety-producing kinds of pleasure first, in order to deal with any apprehensions she may have about them. The pleasuring exercises allow her to do this.

A woman often feels pressured to respond sexually because she is trying to live up to someone else's expectations (those of her partner); she tries to feel something for him instead of for herself, thinking that she must feel aroused or he will be disappointed in her. This of course creates tremendous amounts of anxiety, frustration, depression, and pressure for the woman and is ultimately self-defeating. There is no way that anyone can feel anything for someone else; one can only feel for oneself, because one's feelings are trapped within her own body. If the expectation to respond is removed, and the woman is allowed to feel aroused or not aroused as she desires, the pressure is removed, thus allowing her the opportunity to experience sexual sensations.

STEP 3 BREATHING AND SOUNDS

How: This exercise is for you and your partner to do together and is similar to Step 6 in the previous chapter. If you and your partner don't wish to do this together, skip this step and go on to the next one. Each part of this step should be treated as a separate exercise and should be done on different days.

Part 1: Lie down on the bed side by side on your backs, fully clothed. Imagine that you are in the middle of a sweet-smelling flower garden, and that you are very rested and relaxed. Practice taking deep breaths and letting them out slowly and fully, along with sighing sounds.

When you can both do this easily, continue the same breathing and sighing, but each of you imagine that you are doing something sexual at the same time. Keep doing this until you can both do it naturally and comfortably, and until each thinks the other sounds and looks relaxed.

The next step is to escalate this breathing (without the sexual thoughts) and sighing into a definite noise. The sound should be loud and should rattle through the back of the throat as it comes out. Be careful not to push or force the sound out. Just let it flow out easily and fully.

Imagine that the sound is starting way down in your pelvis, traveling all the way up your windpipe, and rattling through the back of your throat on the way out. *Practice varying the tone and pitch, so that the sound wavers and goes up and down.* Do not screech or scream. Make the sound come out as "ah"; this prevents you from closing off your throat.

Be very careful to breathe as slowly as possible, and to pause a long time between breaths. If you breathe too quickly, you will hyperventilate (upset the balance of oxygen and carbon dioxide in your body), causing dizziness and tingling in the arms, legs, and face. If this happens, slow your breathing as much as possible until the symptoms disappear. Then resume the exercise.

When you can do this exercise so that it sounds and feels relaxed and is easy to do, and when each of you thinks the other person sounds relaxed, continue doing it while imagining that you are doing something sexual. Repeat this until you both can do it naturally and comfortably while thinking sexual thoughts, and until each thinks the other sounds and looks relaxed. If you lose the sexual thoughts, relax as much as possible and then try to re-focus your thoughts.

Part 2: Lie down on the bed side by side on your backs, without any clothes and with the lights on (or in daylight). Begin the deep, slow breathing, along with loud, open, loose "ah" sounds, such as you were doing earlier.

Continue doing this, without any covers or clothes and with the lights on, until you can both do it naturally and comfortably, and until each thinks the other person sounds and looks relaxed.

Now do the same thing while each of you imagines you are doing something sexual. Continue doing this until you can both do it comfortably, and until each thinks the other sounds and looks relaxed.

Part 3: Lie down on the bed side by side on your backs, without any clothes and with the lights on (or in daylight). Begin the deep, slow breathing along with loud, open, loose "ah" sounds, and at the same time *pretend* that you are each masturbating yourself, without the sexual thoughts. Actually make simulated movements of masturbation.

Continue doing this, without any covers or clothes and with the lights on, until you can both do it naturally and comfortably, and until each thinks the other sounds and looks relaxed.

Part 4: Begin this part on the bed without any clothes on, and in full light. The woman is to lie down on the bed on her back, and the man is to lie on top of her in the standard male superior position for intercourse, *without the penis inserted into the vagina.* Both are to begin the deep, slow breathing, along with loud, open, loose "ah" sounds. As you do this, both are to begin movements of intercourse while *pretending* to be having intercourse. The man, being in a better position to move, is to use as much body movement as possible. The woman, although more restricted by her position, should also move as much as she can.

Continue doing this, without any covers or clothes and with the lights on, until you can both do it naturally and comfortably, and until each thinks the other sounds and looks relaxed.

Part 5: Begin this part on the bed without any clothes on, and in full light. The man is to lie down on the bed on his back, and the woman is to sit on top of him in the standard female superior position for intercourse, *without the penis inserted into the vagina.* Both are to begin the deep, slow breathing, along with loud, open, loose "ah" sounds. As you do this, both are to begin movements of intercourse while *pretending* to have intercourse. The woman, being in a better position to move, is to use as much body movement as possible. The man, although more restricted by his position, should also move as much as he can.

Continue doing this, without any covers or clothes and with the lights on, until you can both do it naturally and comfortably, and until each thinks the other sounds and looks relaxed. (Note: If your partner has difficulty doing this exercise, have him refer to the previous chapter and complete Step 6 alone first before doing this step together.)

Part 6: Repeat Steps 3 to 5, this time exaggerating what you feel are the normal sounds and movements as much as possible. Without becoming hysterical, you are to exaggerate your sounds and movements as a bad actor exaggerates a "dying" scene in a Grade B movie.

You may consider this exercise completed when you can both do all the parts naturally and comfortably. This may mean repeating some of the parts on different days before moving on to the next part.

Why: It is very important to feel relaxed during lovemaking if you are to feel aroused. However, it is sometimes difficult to feel comfortable displaying signs of arousal in front of another, since arousal is such a private feeling and something that one cannot really share with someone else, except indirectly. This presents a real dilemma, since intercourse always includes the presence of another person. It is necessary, then, first to practice *simulating* arousal together as a way of testing the reaction of your partner. The final step of exaggeration allows you to actualize your fear of making a "fool" of yourself. After the exaggeration of "role playing," sounds and movements in actual lovemaking seem less threatening. LoPiccolo has reported good results with the use of such "role plays" in treating orgasmic dysfunction.[3]

These exercises will allow you to experience being isolated enough from your partner to concentrate on your own movements, and breathing and sounds, without regard to his opinion about it, and at the same time being intimately involved in coordinating the movement of your bodies together.

Most people find it easy to be concerned about how their partner feels during lovemaking. The real difficulty is being concerned about how *you* feel without regard to your partner. This does not at all mean that you should not be sensitive or loving, but it is impossible for the woman to feel aroused or to experience orgasm if she is worried about what her partner thinks of her "performance."

The objective of this step is to free you from feeling inhibited about sounds and movements in the presence of your partner, without the added stress of actually trying to feel aroused at the same time. When you are able to do Part 6 of this step, you will have accomplished this; the first five parts are merely gradually increasing segments of Part 6, set out in a way that minimizes anxiety by having you accomplish only a small part at a time. This allows you to overcome your anxiety in small stages rather than dealing with large amounts at once. For more information on the importance of breathing and sounds, refer to Step 6 in the previous chapter under *Why*.

Although this exercise should be taken seriously, you may not feel serious as you are doing it. In fact, you both may feel rather ridiculous and end up laughing, especially when you get to the last part of the exercise. This is perfectly normal.

STEP 4 MASTURBATION TOGETHER

How: This exercise is for you and your partner to do together. If you or your partner do not wish to do this together, skip this step and go on to the next one.

This step may be quite difficult for you to do. You or your partner may still feel that there is something wrong about masturbating, especially in front of each other. You may be embarrassed, afraid of so much self-exposure, or of looking foolish. Most people will probably experience at least some of these feelings before beginning this step. In spite of these worries, this is an important exercise to do together. If you are willing to share your feelings of concern with each other, much of the anxiety can be dispelled. The other important ingredient to success here is a sense of humor. You may need to laugh at yourselves a little and not take it all so seriously. This will dispel anxiety and free you from tension so that you can then do the exercise properly.

Part 1: Lie down on the bed side by side *in the dark.* Set a kitchen-type timer or an alarm clock for twenty minutes, but face it and all other clocks or watches in the room away from you. Each of you is to masturbate *yourself* until the timer signals the completion of the exercise. Continue for the entire twenty minutes unless you both have an orgasm before then. Talk during this exercise if you need to, but confine your conversation to sharing feelings about what you are doing. Repeat this two or three times a week until you can *both* reach orgasm in this manner.

Part 2: Lie down on the bed side by side *in full light*, Each of you masturbate *yourself* until the timer signals the completion of the exercise at twenty minutes. Talk during this exercise if you need to, but confine your conversation to your reactions about what you are doing. *Keep your eyes closed* for the duration of the exercise, and continue for the full twenty minutes unless you both have an orgasm before then. Repeat this two or three times a week until you can both reach orgasm in this manner.

Part 3: Lie down on the bed side by side *in full light*. Masturbate *yourselves* until the timer signals the completion of the exercise at twenty minutes. Talk during this exercise if you need to, but confine your conversation to your feelings about what you are doing. *Keep your eyes open without looking at each other* for the duration of the exercise, and continue for the full twenty minutes unless you both have an orgasm before then. Repeat this two or three times a week until you can both reach orgasm in this manner.

Part 4: Lie down on the bed side by side *in full light*. Masturbate *yourselves* until the timer signals the completion of the exercise at twenty minutes unless you both have an orgasm before then. Talk during this exercise if you need to, but confine your conversation to your reaction about what you are doing. *Keep your eyes open and spend most of the time looking at each other*. Repeat this two or three times a week until you can both reach orgasm in this manner.

Part 5: Position yourselves comfortably on the bed, without clothes and *in full light*. You are to masturbate yourself in your usual manner while the man watches and helps you. You should give the major part of the stimulation to yourself. Talk during this exercise if you like, but confine your conversation to your feelings about what you are doing. Continue until you reach orgasm or the timer signals the end of the twenty minutes, whichever occurs first. Repeat this two or three times a week until you can reach orgasm in this manner, but *alternate every other time with Part 6 below*. (Your partner may stimulate himself to orgasm after this exercise if he wishes to.)

Part 6: Position yourselves comfortably on the bed, without clothes and *in full light*. The man is to masturbate himself in his usual manner while you watch and help him. He should give the major part of the stimulation to himself. Talk during this exercise if you like, but confine your conversation to your reactions about what you are doing. Continue until he reaches orgasm or the timer signals the end of the twenty minutes, whichever occurs first. Repeat this two or three times a week until he can reach orgasm in this manner, but *alternate every other time with Part 6 above*. (You may stimulate yourself to orgasm after this exercise if you wish to.) (Note: If either one of you has difficulty doing this step, use breathing and sounds throughout the exercise. It will relax you and help prevent you from holding back on sensations.)

Why: The objective of this step is to free you from feeling inhibited about experiencing arousal and orgasm in the presence of your partner, without the added stress of feeling in any way responsible for his arousal or orgasm.

Most people will be nervous at the thought of this exercise. This is quite understandable, since masturbation is usually considered a private matter. However, it needn't be so, and in fact can add a great amount of variety to the sexual relationship between a man and a woman. In spite of your belief that you could never get through such an exercise, most couples who undergo therapy at the clinic complete this very easily, sometimes to their great surprise. One couple in therapy referred to this exercise as "the last secret."

Once this exercise is completed, the man can feel free to stimulate his own penis during lovemaking if he is losing some of his erection, perhaps from changing positions or from not enough movement; the woman can feel free to stimulate her own genitals when she needs added stimulation. These things, which are sometimes important and necessary parts of successful lovemaking with a partner, could never be done if either person felt inhibited about touching him/herself genitally in front of the other.

There is an additional reason for the woman to do this exercise: experiencing orgasm during intercourse of course requires experiencing orgasm in front of her partner. This can be rather intimidating if thus far you have only experienced orgasms alone during masturbation, and you may feel shy or inhibited about experiencing true arousal and orgasm with your lover present.

For this reason, a transitional step is needed to facilitate the attainment of the goal (orgasm with intercourse). The known stimulation (masturbation) which produces a known response (orgasm) is introduced with the partner present, in order to ensure the greatest possibility of orgasm in a situation which is no longer solitary, but includes the partner. His participation in the exercise greatly diminishes the woman's anxiety over being "watched."

The use of a timer or alarm allows you to avoid looking at the clock and still time the length of the exercise. If you are nervous about the exercise, and many will be, the tendency will be to want to keep checking the clock to see if the time is up (and it can seem to drag on forever if you are doing something unpleasant). But you will be able to involved yourself in the exercise to a greater extent if you are not distracted by checking the time, and you therefore stand to get much more out of the exercise. For this reason it is very important to use the timer each time you do this step.

As with all parts of the instructions in this chapter and the previous one, the final goal of this exercise is approached on a very gradual basis, allowing both of you to overcome small amounts of anxiety at a time rather than large amounts. As you are by now aware, this allows you the best possible opportunity to easily and comfortably accomplish the final goal of the exercise, and your ultimate goal—intercourse resulting in orgasm for both partners. In addition, the likelihood of success is greater if you do the exercise repeatedly in short (twenty-minute) sessions, rather than marathons in which you might feel more frustrated and fatigued.

STEP 5 CLITORAL WITH VAGINAL PUBOCOCCYGEAL STIMULATION

How: This exercise is for you and your partner to do together. If you or your partner do not wish to do it, skip this step and go on to the next one.

This may be done instead of, before, or after intercourse. Precede this with some kind of non-genital touching, such as a body caress. When you are relaxed and ready, set a kitchen-type timer for twenty minutes. Begin masturbating your clitoris in your usual manner, while at the same time your partner stimulates the pubococcygeus muscle in your vagina.

In order for him to locate the muscle, you will need to

squeeze your vagina together several times as he positions his finger to a greater or lesser depth in the vagina. The part that closes against his finger, about a third of the way in, is the muscle. As he stimulates it, let him know if he is touching the part that feels best. You can experiment and concentrate on whatever part feels good to you. Tell him exactly where and how you wish to be stimulated, and when to go faster or slower. Direct him to stimulate you the way you usually do.

Continue this exercise until you have an orgasm, or until the timer goes off at twenty minutes. Do this exercise each time you have love play with your partner, or two or three times a week. You may consider the exercise completed when you can reach orgasm in this manner.

Why: The purpose of this exercise is to begin letting your partner participate in the stimulation which brings you to orgasm. This exercise is essentially what you do when you masturbate, except that your partner is actively involved in part of the stimulation. This enables you to experience having orgasms in his presence, with his help, in a manner which closely resembles that which you are used to, and without the added pressure of trying to please him in any way at the same time. *You* are to take responsibility for seeking your own orgasm by controlling the exercise.

The use of the timer serves the same purpose as in the past: it allows you to relax instead of worrying about whether or not you are taking too much or too little time.

STEP 6 MANUAL CLITORAL STIMULATION BY A PARTNER

How: This exercise is an optional one for you and your partner to do together. If you prefer, skip this step.

After some pleasuring, such as a body caress, begin to masturbate, with your partner present, in your usual manner, except using only clitoral stimulation. As your orgasm begins, give a prearranged signal to your partner, at which point he takes over the stimulation of your clitoris with his hand, trying to duplicate the kind of stroking you were doing. This will require some lengthy discussions about the kind of technique you prefer in order to achieve arousal and orgasm. These talks can be done before, during, and after this exercise, as needed. If you lose the orgasm completely, resume your own stimulation, and again switch to having your partner stimulate you as the orgasm begins. Do this up to three times in one session but for no longer than twenty minutes. If you are unable to complete your orgasm with your partner stimulating you, you may have an orgasm by masturbating yourself if you desire. Continue this process each time you have love play with your partner, or two or three times a week, until you can finish your orgasm with his hand instead of yours stimulating your clitoris.

When you have accomplished the above, move the moment of bringing in his hand further and further from the moment of orgasm. This should be done very gradually over as much time as it takes. Eventually you will reach a point where you will just begin your own stimulation, or where you may respond to stimulation done completely by your partner.

For those women who masturbate using a vibrator, the same method of transmitting the experience to a partner can be used. You simply masturbate in your usual manner with the vibrator (except using only clitoral stimulation). As the orgasm begins, give a prearranged signal to your partner, at which point he takes over the stimulation of your clitoris with his hand, trying to duplicate the kind of stroking you were doing with the vibrator.

Why: There is nothing intrinsically "shameful" about stimulating yourself to arousal or orgasm in the presence of your partner. Since the basic responsibility for your arousal and orgasm lies with you, this is a very direct way to accomplish it. So if you are a woman who has no desire to learn to respond orgasmically to her partner's hand stimulation, skip this step altogether. Stimulating yourself, when you desire direct genital stimulation to arousal or orgasm, is perfectly valid and normal.

However, a great many women will wish to learn to respond orgasmically to their partner's manual stimulation of them. Many of these women will be able to do this without going through this step. But others will have some difficulty translating the experience to a partner, and for these women a gradual transition is required. Small changes are more similar to the original successful technique (self-stimulation) than large changes, and are therefore more likely to allow you to continue having your usual sexual response (orgasm).

STEP 7 USING YOUR VAGINAL PUBOCOCCYGEAL MUSCLE DURING INTERCOURSE

How: This is an exercise that you can easily do without any special cooperation from your partner. There is no requirement for him to do anything, except that you can only practice this during intercourse.

Following some kind of pleasuring, as you are having intercourse, consciously contract (squeeze together) your vagina (pubococcygeus muscle). You may do this each time as the penis is going out, or each time as the penis is going in, as long as you do it regularly and rhythmically. You should hold the squeeze until the penis starts in the other direction, and then rest until it starts back in the direction in which you squeeze it.

Continue this for the duration of intercourse, or for as long as you can if you must stop squeezing before intercourse is completed. If intercourse does not result in the man's ejaculation, the decision to end is up to either one of you. *Do this each time you have intercourse from now on.*

You may consider this exercise completed when you can *easily* squeeze your vaginal muscle during intercourse, with a resultant increase in sensation for you. You may then move on to Step 8, although you will be continuing to squeeze your muscle during intercourse.

Why: The objective of this exercise is to increase vaginal stimulation during intercourse. When you squeeze your vagina, you are stimulating the nerve endings in the pubococcygeus muscle, thus producing pleasant sensations in your vagina. The more stimulation you receive, the greater your arousal. As noted before, this technique is also extremely pleasurable for your partner and in certain cultures is considered an integral part of lovemaking.

Of course, to be able to do this squeezing exercise correctly, you will need to have strength and control of your pubococcygeus muscle. You have to have a substantial muscle to "feel" with, which is why an evaluation by a gynecologist is required.

If you have come this far in the exercises and have neglected to have an examination of the muscle or to do the maintenance exercises once the muscle is in good condition, you should stop and turn back to Part 3, Chapter 1 and review the section on the pubococcygeus muscle, and then turn to Part 3, Chapter 2 and review and do Step 2. Then return to this step and begin it again. This cannot be emphasized enough; unless your muscle is in good physical condition you simply won't have enough nerve endings to feel sensation, and without good strength and control of the muscle, you will be unable to tighten it enough to feel aroused.

STEP 8 MOVEMENTS DURING INTERCOURSE

How: This is an exercise that you can easily do without any special cooperation from your partner. He is not required to do anything, except that you can only practice this during intercourse. However, it is suggested that you try going through the movements alone before you attempt them during intercourse. If you have a steady partner, the two of you can do a "dry run" together while *simulating* intercourse (without the penis inserted). Be prepared to feel somewhat awkward and perhaps a little ridiculous at first.

The movement described below is a little tricky to learn and difficult to describe but, like anything else, fairly simple once you know how. Don't be frustrated if it takes you several attempts to figure it out.

Following some kind of pleasuring, begin intercourse. The action of the penis going in and out of the vagina does very little by itself to stimulate the nerve endings in the pubococcygeus muscle. The surest way of getting this stimulation is to move your hips up and down in a rotating motion (think of a bump and grind), at the same time using your pubococcygeus muscle as described in Step 7. This will cause the penis to rub against your muscle, giving you greatly increased sensation.

If you are lying on your back, bend your knees, bringing your feet to rest soles down on the bed. Using your feet as leverage, raise your pelvis slightly while rotating it in a downward direction. Then relax your pelvis as you move it in an upward direction. This can be done quite comfortably without great effort and requires a minimum of actual movement.

Once you have mastered this pelvic motion, add the squeezing of the pubococcygeus muscle. Squeeze the muscle as you move your pelvis in an upward direction, and relax your muscle as you rotate your pelvis in a downward direction.

If you are on top, insert the penis, and "walk" forward on your knees so that your thighs rest in the indentation of your partner's body just below the ribcage. Then lean forward so that your forearms, with your legs bent, rest on the mattress. If your partner is too large to allow you to do this comfortably, place a pillow under each forearm to elevate yourself. In this position, you can perform the same swivel motion that you did on the bottom, using your knees as leverage. You can also lean backward and forward on your knees without swiveling, still causing penile contact against the twelve o'clock and six o'clock portions of the muscle. This is a particularly good position for those women who experience pain from pressure against the cervix caused by deep thrusting, as the penis is deflected against the vaginal walls rather than inward toward the cervix.

The type of swivel motion described can be used in essentially any position, *provided that you have something to push against with your feet or knees.* In fact, it can just as easily be used by your partner, so the two of you can do this simultaneously, perhaps take turns. (He will find that your movements, as well as his own if he does this, will also greatly increase his stimulation.)

Repeat this on several occasions before going on to Step 8. You may consider this exercise completed when you are confident that you are moving in such a way as to create increased vaginal sensation. *Do this each time you have intercourse from now on.*

Why: The extent to which you move or don't move your own body during intercourse will determine, to a large degree, how much sensation you will feel and whether or not you will experience orgasm.

The objective of this exercise is for you to find ways of moving your pelvis so that the pubococcygeus muscle rubs against the penis during intercourse, which will stimulate and arouse you; and to be able to coordinate this movement with squeezing your vaginal muscle. The more aroused you feel, the greater the likelihood of orgasm.

STEP 9 CLITORAL STIMULATION DURING INTERCOURSE

How: You can only practice this during intercourse, but you need no special cooperation from your partner. *If you have already achieved orgasm during intercourse, skip this step.*

Following foreplay, have intercourse in your usual manner, squeezing your pubococcygeus muscle and moving your pelvis to ensure the greatest amount of vaginal stimulation. At the same time, stimulate your clitoris as you do during masturbation. Try to coordinate the clitoral stimulation with the pelvic movement and the squeezing of the muscle. This may take a little practice.

If you normally masturbate with a vibrator, the best position to use is rear entry (either lying on your abdomen or on your hands and knees, or sideways, the man facing your back—your legs and his should be slightly bent); or you on top facing your partner's feet instead of his face; or lying back on the edge of a "platform" (a lowered or raised bed) while your partner kneels or stands facing you.

Continue doing this until you have an orgasm, or until intercourse ends by mutual agreement or your partner's ejaculation, whichever occurs first. Each time you have intercourse, repeat this in a position which allows for clitoral stimulation, until you can easily have an orgasm in this manner.

A variation of this step is clitoral stimulation during intercourse provided by the man. (This is best done after having successfully completed Step 6, Manual Genital Stimulation by a Partner.) The process is as described above except that the man stimulates your clitoris throughout intercourse. This partner-stimulation can be alternated with self-stimulation if desired.

Why: The objective of this step is to duplicate the sensations of masturbation as closely as possible, thus increasing the likelihood of orgasm.

The combination of clitoral stimulation, squeezing the pubococcygeus muscle and rotating your pelvis to allow full penile contact against and stimulation of the muscle is almost a duplication of the kind of stimulation that you receive during masturbation when it produces orgasm. By practicing, you can re-create those same feelings with intercourse, thus eventually reaching orgasm.

By now you are probably beginning to understand that you must actively seek and work for your own orgasm, just as your partner does. The more you practice, the sooner it will happen. But there is no need to rush or to pressure yourself. Just keep doing the exercises (Steps 7, 8 and 9) each time you have intercourse. As long as you are having intercourse anyway, you might just as well be working toward your own satisfaction, even if it takes a few months to achieve it.

STEP 10 TAPERING OFF CLITORAL STIMULATION DURING INTERCOURSE

How: This is an exercise you can do without any special cooperation from your partner. You can only practice it during intercourse, however.

The process of tapering off clitoral stimulation during intercourse is similar to tapering off vibrator masturbation. But this should only be done if you are able to attain orgasm easily during intercourse with concurrent clitoral stumulation. *If you do not wish to taper off clitoral stimulation during intercourse,* skip this step.

Following some kind of pleasuring, such as a body caress, have intercourse, squeezing your vaginal muscle and moving your pelvis to ensure the greatest amount of vaginal stimulation, and using clitoral stimulation at the same time. As your orgasm begins, continue having intercourse, but stop the clitoral stimulation. If you lose the orgasm completely, resume clitoral stimulation immediately, and again stop the clitoral stimulation as your orgasm begins. Do this up to three times in one lovemaking session, and if you are unable to complete your orgasm without clitoral stimulation, you may have an orgasm with concurrent clitoral stimulation if you so desire. Continue doing this each time you have intercourse until you can easily complete your orgasm without clitoral stimulation.

When you have accomplished the above, move the moment of stopping the clitoral stimulation further and further from the point of orgasm. This should be done very gradually over as much time as it takes. Eventually you will reach a point where you will just begin intercourse with clitoral stimulation, or where you may not need it at all, or perhaps only as a prelude to intercourse.

It is frequently easier for a woman to experience orgasm during intercourse when she is on top. If she leans down so that her chest is against her partner's chest, he can pull her toward him by firmly grasping her buttocks. This firm pressure sometimes creates additional clitoral stimulation by means of rubbing against the man's pubic bone, and increases the likelihood of orgasm.

If possible, have intercourse two or three times a week during this tapering-off process. The normal period of time required to accomplish a complete switch from intercourse *with* clitoral stimulation to intercourse *without* clitoral stimulation is several weeks. You may consider this step completed when you can easily achieve orgasm during intercourse without concurrent clitoral stimulation.

Why: There is nothing wrong, second-rate, or abnormal about using clitoral stimulation during intercourse. In fact, it produces a significant amount of additional stimulation that is not present in the "no hands" kind of arousal and orgasm with penile stimulation alone. For this reason, many women will wish to continue using clitoral stimulation. If you can reach orgasm during intercourse with concurrent clitoral stimulation and you are satisfied with this method, do not attempt to make a change. You are perfectly normal, and your method of achieving orgasm is perfectly normal.

However, it is true that a great many women are determined to achieve orgasm during intercourse without using their hands. For these women, this method of tapering off hand stimulation will prove helpful. This is especially true when the woman's partner reacts judgmentally to the fact that she needs clitoral stimulation, or for the woman who is in a situation where she may not have the same partner each time she has intercourse, thus causing her to perhaps feel self-conscious about needing clitoral stimulation.

The method of gradually stopping the clitoral stimulation further and further from the point of orgasm is recommended because you are only trying to change a small part of your technique at a time. Small changes are more similar to the original successful technique than large changes, and are more likely to allow you to continue having your usual sexual response.

Note: Because of the variables involved in a relationship, it is more difficult for a woman to successfully learn to be orgasmic with intercourse than with masturbation. If you have carefully followed the steps as recommended and are not having orgasms with intercourse, you may have one of several problems.

Perhaps your pubococcygeus muscle is unhealthy. A visit to a gynecologist for an examination can determine whether you need a medically supervised physical therapy program. Once the physical problem is corrected, the program can be resumed at the beginning of this chapter, assuming you are already orgasmic with masturbation. (If you are unable to have orgasms with masturbation, an unhealthy pubococcygeus muscle is not the problem.)

Perhaps you have not had enough frequency of contact with a partner to build up any momentum. If this is the case, you haven't "failed" the learning program at all—yours wasn't a valid test. You are advised to continue masturbating according to the instructions in Step 11 of the previous chapter on a regular basis of perhaps three to sixteen times a month. In addition, you should not worry about your lack of orgasm with intercourse until you are able to engage in it more frequently. In fact, regular masturbation may be all you need in order to eventually begin having orgasm during intercourse. If you are a shy person, learn to meet and relate to others. Psychotherapy could help you become more outgoing, assertive, and comfortable with others. When your frequency of sexual contact increases, you can begin over again the program outlined in this chapter.

You may be in an ongoing relationship in which your needs are not being met. Perhaps you don't trust your partner or you feel insecure in some way; you may fear that he will leave you for someone else; you may not feel loved in the way you need to; you may not love him but are only pretending to. In this case, psychiatric care aimed at understanding and resolving the conflicts may be a prerequisite to having orgasms in intercourse.

Possibly you only followed the instructions half-heartedly and not very conscientiously, in which case you could simply begin the program over again. In fact, you can do this if you wish regardless of the reason.

There may be psychological problems that are keeping you from responding fully. If this is the case, it is virtually impossible to determine the sources of the problem without help from a psychotherapist. If there are deep unconscious blocks preventing you from experiencing orgasm, the best advice for you is to enter psychotherapy and try to discover what these hidden reasons are.

Finally, it is important to recognize that a large number of perfectly normal and emotionally healthy women do not experience orgasm. The absence of orgasmic response does not mean that there is anything "wrong" with you. A woman can be a perfectly satisfactory, exciting sexual partner without being orgasmic. She can be warm, loving, responsive, desirable, sexy, sensitive, perceptive, interesting, vital, companionable, attractive and feminine without ever having orgasms. She can also be deeply loved and accepted by her partner without having orgasms.

SUMMARY OF THE TEN-STEP PROGRAM FOR ACHIEVING ORGASM WITH INTERCOURSE

Step One

1. Take a bath together and wash and dry each other all over.

2. In another room, sit facing each other, without clothes and in comfortable positions.

3. Take the other's hands in yours and, starting at the head and working downward, show him/her exactly

where and how you like to be touched, using words to explain clearly.

4. Your partner should tell you that he/she understands, while at the same time demonstrating with his hands.

5. As soon as you are both satisfied that he/she understands how you like to be touched in that area, switch roles—it's the other person's turn.

6. Continue alternating back and forth until all nongenital areas of both your bodies have been touched. Then do the genitals and breasts.

7. Take as small an area of the body each time as possible.

8. The object of the exercise is for each of you to take active responsibility in discovering what you like, and to communicate that to your partner.

Step Two

1. Decide who will be the giver and who the receiver.

2. In comfortable positions, using lubricant, one touches the other slowly and lightly while making solid contact with the other's skin.

3. Do this in such a way as to pleasure *yourself*.

4. Practice giving and receiving a facial caress, a body caress without genitals, and a body caress with genitals.

5. Do *not* go on to additional sexual contact at the end of each exercise.

6. After each exercise, share your feelings with each other about what you would have liked, and what you did like.

Step Three

1. Together, fully clothed, practice deep breathing along with sighing sounds. Add a sexual thought to the

breathing and sighing. Continue the breathing, but change the sighing into a loose, free, easy, naturally flowing *loud* "ah" sound that rattles out of the throat. Continue doing this while thinking about something sexual.

2. Together, without clothes in full light, make the loud "ah" sounds as above, along with deep breathing. Add to this a sexual thought.

3. Together, without clothes in full light, make the loud "ah" sounds and breathe while pretending to masturbate yourselves, without the sexual thoughts.

4. Together, without clothes in full light, make the loud "ah" sounds as above, along with deep breathing, in the male superior position for *simulated* intercourse. Move freely throughout.

5. Together, without clothes in full light, make the loud "ah" sounds as above, along with deep breathing, in the female superior position for *simulated* intercourse. Move freely throughout.

6. Repeat Steps 3 to 5, greatly exaggerating your "normal" sounds and movements. Repeat until you and your partner feel comfortable doing this.

Step Four

1. Together in the dark, with eyes open or closed, masturbate *yourselves* for twenty minutes. Repeat this two or three times a week until you can both reach orgasm in this manner.

2. Together in full light, but with your eyes closed, masturbate *yourselves* for twenty minutes. Repeat this two or three times a week until you can both reach orgasm in this manner.

3. Together in full light, with your eyes open but not looking at each other, masturbate *yourselves* for twenty minutes. Repeat this two or three times a week until you can both reach orgasm in this manner.

4. Together in full light, with your eyes open and looking at each other, masturbate *yourselves* for twenty minutes. Repeat this two or three times a week until you can both reach orgasm in this manner.

5. In full light, with your eyes open and looking at each other, the *woman masturbates herself* while the man watches and gives her a small amount of help. Continue for twenty minutes. Repeat two or three times a week until she can reach orgasm in this manner, but *alternate every other time with Step 6 below*.

6. In full light, with your eyes open and looking at each other, the *man masturbates himself* while the woman watches and gives him a small amount of help. Continue for twenty minutes. Repeat two or three times a week until he can reach orgasm in this manner, but *alternate every other time with Step 5 above*.

Step Five

1. Begin with some non-genital touching, such as a body caress.

2. When you feel ready, begin masturbating yourself (only on the clitoris) in your usual manner, while you direct your partner to provide stimulation of the pubococcygeus muscle.

3. Do this for twenty minutes two or three times a week, until you can reach orgasm in this manner.

Step Six

1. After pleasuring, masturbate yourself (only with clitoral stimulation) in your usual manner with your partner present.

2. As your orgasm begins, give a prearranged signal to your partner, at which time he takes over the stimulation of your clitoris with his hand, duplicating the kind of

stroking you were doing as closely as possible. Do this up to three times in one session.

3. Continue this each time you have loveplay until you can easily finish your orgasm with your partner manually stimulating your clitoris.

4. From then on each time you have loveplay, gradually move the moment of bringing in your partner's stimulation of your clitoris further and further from the point of orgasm.

5. Continue this practice each time you have loveplay, or two or three times a week, for as long as it takes to learn to respond orgasmically to manual stimulation by your partner.

Step Seven

1. During intercourse, squeeze your pubococcygeus muscle together as the penis is going out, or as it is going in.

2. Hold the squeeze until the penis starts in the other direction, and then relax.

3. As it starts back in the original direction, squeeze and hold until it starts to go the other way again.

4. Continue doing this rhythmically and regularly until intercourse is completed, or as long as you can.

5. Do this from now on every time you have intercourse.

Step Eight

1. During intercourse, move your pelvis in a swivel motion against the penis, while at the same time squeezing your vaginal muscle.

2. Do this each time you have intercourse from now on in those positions which allow this movement.

Step Nine

1. During intercourse, while squeezing your vagina and swiveling your pelvis, stimulate your clitoris as you do during masturbation, or have your partner stimulate your clitoris.

2. Continue doing this until you have an orgasm or until intercourse ends, whichever occurs first.

3. Repeat this each time you have intercourse in a position which allows for clitoral stimulation, until you can easily have an orgasm in this manner.

Step Ten

1. Following pleasuring, have intercourse in your usual manner, squeezing your vaginal muscle, moving your pelvis, and giving yourself clitoral stimulation.

2. As your orgasm begins, stop the clitoral stimulation but continue having intercourse (the vaginal stimulation).

3. Continue this each time you have intercourse until you can easily finish your orgasm with vaginal stimulation alone.

4. From then on each time you have intercourse, gradually move the moment of stopping the clitoral stimulation further and further from the point of orgasm.

5. Have intercourse two or three times a week if possible for as long as it takes fully to taper off direct clitoral stimulation during intercourse.

PART 4

The Road to the Future

Sexuality in the past has been obscured by superstition, arbitrary morality, and ignorance. It is not surprising that, in the minds of many, female orgasmic difficulties became associated with mental illness, immaturity, and emotional instability.

Many now believe that a sexual revolution has occurred and that such attitudes are outdated. Experience at the clinic and elsewhere has shown that in fact sexual revolution is a myth. Although there is much more "sex" in advertising, movies, and literature, people's underlying sexual attitudes are still inhibiting their behavior. This is commonly seen even in young people who, although statistics indicate they are beginning activity at an earlier age, are appearing at the clinic and elsewhere with the same sexual problems as their parents. This is really not so surprising as it might at first seem, because they really have not received any better preparation for a satisfactory sex life than their parents did.

Hopefully this book has helped you with your difficulties. But what about your daughter or your granddaughter? What about the female child as yet unborn? Can her life be directed in such a way that she does not have to undergo the years of shame and ignorance that have become the burden of so many women? Can preventive medicine be practiced in this all-important area of human functioning?

The answer to these questions is an emphatic *yes*. The key to the prevention of sexual dysfunction is adequate sex education. Unfortunately, there currently exists a serious gap in sex education. It is true that medical science and psychology have developed in the last fifty years an impressive and extensive body of knowledge about human sexuality. But in spite of such works as gynecologist R. L. Dickinson's and Lura Beam's *A Thousand Marriages*, in which they followed the sexual life cycles of his patients from childhood through menopause;[1] the statistical studies of Kinsey; and the research of Masters and Johnson, the general population remains woefully uneducated in sexual matters. This gap between knowledge and education has caused much of today's sexual unhappiness.

Historically, sexual knowledge has been kept from people in a vain attempt to control sexual functioning itself. As Bertrand Russell put it in *Marriage and Morals:*

"It was at first only females who were to be kept ignorant. . . . Gradually, however, women acquiesced in the view that ignorance is essential to virtue, and partly through their influence it came to be thought that children and young people, whether male or female, should be as ignorant as possible on sexual subjects. At this stage the motive . . . passed into the region of irrational taboo."[2]

The Sex Information and Education Council of the United States (SIECUS) explains at some length how the avoidance of sex education is an educational process all its own:

"Most people assume that, in the absence of direct

instruction, no sex education takes place. Actually, the parents' reaction to themselves and to each other as sexual beings, their feelings toward the child's exploration of his own body, their method of establishing the child's toilet habits, their response to his questions and his attempts to learn about himself and his environment, their ability to give and express their love for each other and for him, are among the many ways in which they profoundly influence the child's sexual conditioning. Avoidance, repression, rejection, suppression, embarrassment, and shock are negative forms of sex education. That fact cannot be escaped. Parents cannot choose whether or not they will give sex education; they can choose only whether they will do something positive or negative about it, whether they will accept or deny the responsibility."[8]

The adult woman of today has had to learn as an adult what she should have been taught as a child and should have learned as an adolescent. Before she can learn successfully as an adult, however, she must go through the difficult process of *unlearning* the negative sex attitudes from her upbringing. This makes her task much more formidable than it would have been as a child and adolescent. Therefore, it is incumbent upon every parent to provide his or her children with adequate sexual knowledge, presented in a positive manner, in order to prevent later sexual trauma. Both fathers and mothers must share in this responsibility.

What is needed in the area of prevention is knowledge and specific practical guidelines for parents. In an attempt to respond to this need, we present here the questions most frequently asked at the clinic by parents and our answers to these questions.

At what age should sex education begin?

Sex education always begins in infancy whether the parents consciously educate the baby or not. In order for this education to be positive rather than negative, certain guidelines are recommended. Genital touching and exploration should be allowed within the bounds of privacy right from the start, and should continue to be allowed throughout puberty. Self-exploration and exploration of other children is a natural process observed in many animals and many cultures and is perfectly normal. It is a necessary process for the development of a positive body image, which is so important in successful sexual functioning later in life. Indeed, histories of both male and female patients at the clinic show that punishment for early childhood genital play is often one of the causes of sexual dysfunction.

G.G. was seen for primary orgasmic dysfunction (she had never had an orgasm) and lack of sexual satisfaction. She recounted how for many years she had been aware that she was simply unable to touch her genitals in spite of a desire to do so. She was completely unable to masturbate as an adult, although she wanted to. She told the therapists that she had been in psychotherapy for many years before her therapist uncovered an incident from early childhood that provided insight into her problem. In the patient's own words: "My mother came to take care of me when the burden of my problem became so great I was unable to function. She had a session with my therapist and with reluctance revealed that she had caught me touching myself at age three and severely punished me. I don't remember the incident at all."

There is no set time for giving specific sexual information. The time for simple, honest answers is when the questions are asked. Hesitation or evasion of questions instead of a simple, honest answer creates anxiety in the child.

Parents often make the mistake of trying to be too inclusive in response to a child's question. For example:

Child: "Where did I come from?"

Parent: (Goes into a ten-minute description of intercourse and reproduction.)

Child: "Yes, but where did I come from?"

Obviously it is wise to understand just what it is your child wants to know before going into a dissertation-like answer. When a child of three asks where babies come from, it is totally unnecessary and confusing to attempt an entire explanation of reproductive biology. Often a simple answer such as: "A baby comes from its mother and father" is enough. If it is not, the child will continue to question you, and you can continue to answer until she is satisfied for that moment. The attitude in which you respond is of much greater significance than the quantity of information expressed.

Although there is no set time for teaching your child about sex, as a general rule no child should have to be faced with the hormonal surges of puberty before fully understanding human sexual functioning.

Should sex education come from the school, the church, or the home?

It should come from all three. Unfortunately, today's religious and educational systems are inadequate in this regard, with very few exceptions. And, unhappily, many parents lack knowledge of the subject. In many instances sex education is rigidly controlled by laws, and there does not seem to be much hope at present that the public school system will be able to provide adequate sex education in the face of these rigid controls. In California a former governor consistently vetoed liberal sex education bills for years, and the Educational Code has provided strict rules in regard to sex education. Recently a school superintendent in southern California lost his job for permitting a liberal sex education program in his school district, even though it was desired by the majority of parents.

Parents must help by putting strong pressure on their schools (especially through P.T.A.) and their legislators for sex education for both adults and children. But a parent's main responsibility today is to provide a home atmosphere in which sex education is positive in order to counteract any negative sex instruction that may be obtained from school, church, and friends.

Fortunately, many religious leaders are adopting a more liberal approach to sex education, and often the religious school can provide an adjunct to home education. But it must be emphasized that this is by no means universally true, and parents must carefully examine the attitudes of the religious leaders with whom their children are entrusted. Religious orthodoxy has provided the breeding ground for some of the most serious sexual problems seen at the clinic, and continues to do so.

The final responsibility for positive sex education still rests with the parents.

What if my child never asks me any questions about sex?

Any child who is not raised in a vacuum will have a great deal of curiosity about sex. If she doesn't ask you, it is probably because she feels she can't or shouldn't. In either case, her reluctance stems from an attitude about sex which she has picked up from you. By age three children should be asking some questions about where babies come from, and the questions should continue from there. If you notice that your child never asks questions, re-evaluate what *you* are doing to create this situation. Perhaps talk to some friends about it, or see a therapist to explore the issue. In any case, begin talking to your child to find out what she wants to know. Be honest with her and you will get honest answers.

What if the child walks in during lovemaking?

An attitude of calmness and naturalness is important. If the child is severely punished or even reprimanded for viewing a sexual act, she will become convinced that the act itself is wrong. However, it must be stressed that parents have a right to privacy. Bedroom doors should be locked, not to punish the children but to allow uninterrupted intimate time for adults. If a child is curious about this privacy, her questions should be answered honestly. Children should be told that Mommy and Daddy need special time alone to love each other in private. Again, further questions should be answered simply and honestly.

Should children be exposed to adult nudity?

The naked body is a reality and also a thing of artistic beauty. In many cultures, nudity is common. Yet many adults persist in regarding the naked body with shame. They quickly cover themselves when the child approaches.

Again, the parent's general attitude is more important than any specific rule. Nudity occurs naturally at many points in the day and should be treated naturally. If it is, the child will inevitably be at least occasionally exposed to it, and nudity will be a natural, non-traumatic experience for her.

What if I am too embarrassed to answer my child's questions?

There are only two things that any responsible adult can do in this situation. First of all, be honest with your child about your discomfort. Either tell her that you would like to discuss these things with her but that you aren't used to talking about sex and don't feel comfortable enough to answer her questions; or try to answer what questions you can in spite of your discomfort, at the same time admitting your embarrassment to her. Discussions about sex do get easier with practice. Secondly, always make provisions for her to talk to someone if she can't talk to you—a friend of the family, a teacher, a doctor—but somebody whom she can relate to easily and who can give her accurate information. Meanwhile, educate yourself so that you become more and more comfortable in discussing sex. This can be done by taking formal classes which are offered in some colleges and universities. Or, if these are not available, by organizing your own with your friends or through your church or social group and inviting community professionals to conduct them. As you learn more, you can begin to share this knowledge with your child, and communicating about sex will gradually become easier and more comfortable.

What if my child asks me things I can't answer?

She will. Your only responsibilities are to be honest in telling her that you don't know, and to try to provide a way for her to find out. Again, you can guide her toward someone who is more of an authority—the family doctor, a nurse, a teacher—who can simply tell her the information she wishes to know. If she is too embarrassed to ask, find out for her and tell her the answer. Or go to the library together and research the answer. You may have to be creative to find out what she wants to know, but your willingness to make an effort will be one of the most positive steps you can make in sexually educating your child.

How old should a girl be when she begins sexual activity?

The age at which young people begin sexual activity in general is earlier now than in the past.[4] However, even young people seem to have set a limit as to how young is "too young." Teenage "rap" groups at Planned Parenthood clinics have provided some surprising insights. After an initial period in which the teenagers' gripes about the restrictions placed on them by their parents are explored, they are asked how they would react if their twelve-year-old daughter came home and asked if she could have intercourse with her boyfriend in her bedroom. The teenagers usually reply: "Twelve years old? Ridiculous!" or: "Not in my house!" It would appear that any age younger than when you started seems too early. In these children, the parental conditioning has already taken root, and even though they themselves feel oppressed, they are prone to oppress their own children.

Mary Calderone has noted that children experience sexual feelings very early; in fact, some even experience what appears to be orgasm as early as the first year.[5] Childhood sexuality is a reality that cannot be denied. When this normal sex play changes to "for real" is inconsequential. What is important is that children be provided with adequate education about venereal disease and contraception as a natural process of learning. When a child passes through puberty and is able to conceive, then contraception should be easily available upon request. To react any differently, to debate issues of morality while denying reality, is sheer folly. In fact, the young person who has extensive information about all aspects of sexual functioning is *less* likely to engage in casual or promiscuous sexual behavior than is her more ignorant peer. Young persons should be neither discouraged nor encouraged to engage in sex activities, but merely educated. Education in the broadest sense means two-way conversations with your child on the consequences, both emotional and physical, of sexual activity. It also means honesty from you, the parent—presenting your biases but stating them as such. If you truly believe that sex before marriage is wrong, or you are uncomfortable about the idea, say so and discuss it together—but don't try to use your feelings to control your child's sexual behavior. Any attempt would likely be in vain, since she will undoubtedly carry out sexual activities without your knowledge while acquiescing verbally to your views. She must make her decisions for herself, and you can help her most by being available to discuss problems as they arise. This requires an honest relationship in which you know what she is doing even if you don't feel comfortable about her doing it.

You must also be willing to hear what your child is really saying ("I do or I don't want to have sex") and to help *her* ascertain what she is saying and feeling, and why.

In summary, each child must be free to decide for herself when and whether she will begin sexual activity. The responsibility of the parent is to guide the girl away from situations which are likely to harm her either emotionally or physically. (Sex with a partner who has syphilis, or sex without contraception can create physical harm; sex with someone who is married to another, or sex with someone much older can create emotional harm.) A decision not to engage in sexual activities at all or until marriage must be respected and honored as much as the decision to have sex early. The job of guiding one's child is a difficult one at best, and can only be done effectively if there is open, honest, loving communication and respect between parent and child.

What kinds of toys and books for children are recommended for preventing sex-stereotyped upbringing?

The devastating effect of role-constricting upbringing has been a major thesis of this book. The concept of little boys and little girls as different species, raised and treated in totally different ways, accounts for much of the sexual misery of today. The entrapment of men and women into sex-stereotyped roles is a major cause of sexual problems in our society.

Toys and books should not foster a passive-dependent role for girls or an aggressive, over-responsible role for boys. Little girls should be allowed and encouraged to have rough-and-tumble play and not be labeled as tomboys, but they should also be allowed and encouraged to use traditional girls' toys as well. Little boys should be allowed and encouraged to play with dolls and with homemaking toys, but they should also be allowed and encouraged to use traditional boys' toys. In other words, children of both sexes should be exposed to a wide range of toys so they can feel free to pick those which appeal to their interests, and their interests should be fostered in a direction that is not confined to stereotypes.

Parents should avoid traditional fairy tales and children's stories that stereotype female (and male) roles, such as *Sleeping Beauty* and *Cinderella*. If such stories are read, they should be followed by a discussion of these roles and of ways in which the characters in the stories might have acted instead of how they did act. Another alternative is to read traditional stories, but to change the ending so that the female heroines are portrayed as actively taking responsibility for their lives. This is particularly effective with very young children who cannot read. With older children, parents can simply tell their children that they like the story their way and that is why they are changing it.

Ms. magazine frequently publishes suggestions of children's books that are not sex-role stereotyped. But the best stories can come from the parents themselves. Children generally like parent-told stories much more than those from books anyway, and this is a marvelous way of communicating parental philosophy to a child in a manner that is appealing rather than lecturing. Stories are a positive teaching aid, and parents should use them to help their children grow. Additional benefits are the pleasure and feeling of intimacy which the parent experiences from communicating creatively with his or her child in this way.

A modification of this approach is to have "family stories" in which two or more persons in the family, including children, take turns making up and telling one continuous story. In this way the child has an opportunity to create any type of role she desires for the characters in the story and isn't bound by predetermined stereotypes. If she has difficulty in doing this—in creating, for instance, active, assertive roles for female characters—she can be helped by the parent who simply takes over the telling of the story for a while until such a character is created, and then turns it back to the child. This process, if repeated, will gradually teach even those children who have been raised within a stereotyped concept of male-female roles to think more freely about activities and behavior as they apply to either sex. This awareness will be incorporated into their own lives and the ways in which they think of themselves; and once such an awareness is created, it should be fostered tenderly but persistently by the parents.

Parents must remain on the alert for toys that are packaged in such a way as to reinforce the stereotypes. If a football you have bought for your little girl comes in a package showing only boys on the box, take it out of the box and re-wrap it before giving it to her. Do the same thing before giving it to a boy, or he too will make the subconscious assumption that football is only for boys, without even knowing why he believes it. Do the same thing with toys that are traditionally "feminine." Unless a package shows both boys and girls equally participating in the activity portrayed, do not expose the child to the package. Many toys, for example, show a boy or boys on the package actively playing some rough or exciting game, with a girl on the sidelines watching. This is an extremely negative message, implying that girls have their place, which isn't anywhere near the action or the fun, and that they derive pleasure not from participating in the game, but from passively watching the boys. (This is what often happens during sexual relations after they become adults.) This message is very discouraging to a girl, who is as likely as a boy to want to participate in what is going on, and fosters in her a passive, dependent attitude, as well as fostering a dominant, superior attitude in boys.

Ms. Foundation's record and book, *Free to Be You and Me,* is an excellent gift for the younger child, since it avoids role stereotypes and creates an atmosphere of freedom of choice based on desire rather than on dictum. It presents stories such as "William Wants a Doll" and the fable of Atlantis—in which a young girl outraces the boys in the kingdom.

In general, however, it is unrealistic to expect that the advertising world will provide non-stereotyped material for children. As a parent, your challenge is to create, improvise, and control your child's toys, books, and activities, and thereby her sexual attitudes.

What specific sex-education materials do you recommend?

An important beginning is the education of the adult. The starred items in the bibliography are recommended for adults. An excellent book is *What to Tell Your Child About Sex* prepared by the Child Study Association of America. This book provides recommended reading for children at different ages. The previously mentioned *Free to Be You and Me* from the Ms. Foundation is excellent for sex-role education. SIECUS, in an appendix to *Sexuality and Man*, provides a list of suggested films and audiovisual aids for different age groups.

For women, the road from the past was a chronicle of how their birthright to sexual happiness was taken from them. The present, including this book, is engaged in an attempt at reclaiming that birthright for women. The road to the future belongs to your children, but you are largely responsible for their success in enjoying sex. Guide them well.

NOTES

PART 1
1. Masters and Johnson (1966), p. 133.
2. Masters and Johnson (1966), p. 133.
3. Masters and Johnson (1966), p. 118.

PART 2
Chapter 1
1. Burns (1961), pp. 76-158.
2. Masters and Johnson (1966), pp. 3-8.
3. Masters and Johnson (1966), p. 69.

Chapter 2
1. Brown (1966), pp. 164–174.
2. Fisher (1973), p. 6.
3. Freud (1955), pp. 3–64.
4. Wright (1953).
5. Masters and Johnson (1966), pp. 137–185.
6. Masters and Johnson (1970), p. 4.
7. Huxley (1954), p. 12.
8. Bergler and Kroger (1954), p. 82.
9. Masters and Johnson (1966), p. 65.
   Sherfey (1966), p. 104.
10. Freud (1938), Vol. 18, pp. 613–614.

11. Bergler and Kroger (1954).
    Bonaparte (1953).
    Bychowski (1949).
    Deutsch (1946).
    Eissler (1939), pp. 191–210.
    Fenichel (1945).
    Hitschmann and Bergler (1949), pp. 45–53.
    Lundberg and Farnham (1967).
12. Robinson (1959).
    Robinson (1959), p. 75.
13. Fisher (1973), pp. 16, 4.
14. Sherfey (1966), p. 47.
15. Freud (1955), Vol. 18, pp. 3–64.
16. Masters and Johnson (1966), p. 67.
17. Masters and Johnson (1966), p. 60.
18. Sherfey (1966), p. 85.
19. Masters and Johnson (1966).
20. Krantz (7:1973).
    Kegel (1952), p. 521.
21. Kaplan (1974), p. 28.
22. Kaplan (1974), p. 29.
23. Kaplan (1974), p. 377.
24. Sherfey (1966), p. 131.
25. Kegel (1952), p. 522.
    McGuire and Steinhilber (1964), p. 418.
26. Achilles (1923).
    Bromley and Britten (1938).
    Davis (1929).
    Hughes (12: 1926), pp. 261–273.
    Pearl (1925).
    Peck and Wells (1925), pp. 502–520.
    Terman (1938).
27. Oliven (1965), p. 465.
    Masters and Johnson (1966), p. 135.
28. Hastings (1969), p. 57.
29. Sherfey (1966), p. 26.
30. Kinsey (1953), p. 628.
31. Hastings (1966), p. 57.
32. Kinsey (1948), p. 59.
33. Kinsey (1953), p. 628.
34. Hunt (1974).

35. Fisher (1973), p. 204.
36. Van de Velde (1930), pp. ix–x.
37. Pomeroy (1972), p. 182.
38. Pomeroy (1972), p. 182.
    Kleegman (1969), p. 24.

Chapter 3
 1. Harlow (1965), pp. 234–265.
    Neiger (1969), pp. 58–61.
 2. Becker (1973), pp. 113–115.
 3. Neiger (1973), p. 61.
 4. Meade (1973), p. 24.
 5. Money (1972), pp. 118–122.
 6. Meade (1973), p. 24.
 7. Sherfey (1966).
 8. Kinsey (1953), p. 173.
 9. Kinsey (1953), p. 138.
10. Kinsey (1953), p. 139.
11. Kinsey (1953), p. 373.
12. Maxwell (1:1973), p. 193.
13. Deutsch (1968), p. 97.
14. Mead (1949), p. 219.
15. Ford and Beach (1951), p. 270.
    LoPiccolo and Lobitz (1972), p. 15.

PART 3
Chapter 1
 1. Kegel (1952), pp. 35–51.
    Kegel (1952).
 2. Kegel (1952), p. 522.
 3. Kegel (1952), p. 522.
 4. Kegel (1952), p. 522.
 5. Comfort (1961), p. 109.
 6. Deutsch (1968), p. 74.
 7. Dickinson (1949).
 8. Van de Velde (1930).
 9. Kegel (1952), p. 523
10. Kegel (1952), p. 523.
11. Oliven (1965), p. 458.
12. Oliven (1965), p. 340.
    Landis (1950), pp. 676–777.

          Terman (1938).
          Rainwater (1965).
          Guttmacher (1970), p. 116.
13. Potts and Peel (1970), p. 105.
14. Guttmacher (1970), p. 20.
15. Kane (1970), pp. 443–450.
16. Clark (1968), p. 154.
17. Clark (1968), p. 154.
18. Seaman (1972), p. 248.
19. Clark (1968), p. 145.
20. Comfort (1972), p. 55.
21. Oliven (1965), pp. 339–340.
22. Masters and Johnson (1966), p. 233.
23. Masters and Johnson (1970), p. 339.
24. Masters and Johnson (1966), p. 57.
25. Graber and Kline-Graber (1974).
26. Clark (1968), p. 17.
27. Oliven (1965), p. 265.
28. Rathmann (1959), p. 116.
29. Clark (1963).
30. Sherfey (1966), p. 131.
31. Wolfe (21:1974), p. 6.
32. Oliven (1965), p. 265.
33. Kaplan (1972), p. 346.
34. Rathmann (1959).
35. Oliven (1965).
36. Semmens (1973), p. 169.
37. Kegel (1952), pp. 521–524.
38. Masters and Johnson (1970), p. 271.
39. Masters and Johnson (1970), p. 268.
40. Oliven (1965), pp. 232–233.

Chapter 2
 1. Masters and Johnson (1966), pp. 227, 240.
          Kaplan (1974), pp. 374–375.
          LoPiccolo and Lobitz (1972), pp. 163–171.
 2. LoPiccolo and Lobitz (1971), pp. 163–171.
 3. LoPiccolo and Lobitz (1971), p. 165.
          Kaplan (1974), p. 388.
 4. Kaplan (1974), p. 388.
 5. Dearborn (1961), p. 204.

6. Hunt (1974), pp. 66–67.
7. Kinsey (1953), p. 166.
8. Tissot (1764), XXIV.
9. Brecher (1969), p. 85.
10. Greenbank (1961), pp. 989–992.
11. Sex Information and Education Council of the United States (1970), p. 67.
12. Kinsey (1948), p. 167.
    Hunt (1974), pp. 76, 85.
13. Ford and Beach (1951).
14. Huxley (1954), p. 12.
15. Comfort (1972), pp. 125–127.
16. LoPiccolo and Lobitz (1973), p. 165.
17. Wolpe (1969).
18. Fisher (1973), p. 55.
19. Lowen (1961), p. 38.
20. SIECUS (1970), p. 69.
21. Fisher (1973), pp. 86–89.
22. Kaplan (1974), p. 390.
23. Kaplan (1974), p. 390.
24. LoPiccolo and Lobitz (2:1972), p. 17.

Chapter 3
1. LoPiccolo, personal communication.
2. Masters and Johnson (1970), p. 187.
3. LoPiccolo and Lobitz (1973).
4. Kaplan (1974), pp. 391, 452.
   Kegel (1952), pp. 521–524.

PART 4
1. Dickinson (1931).
2. Russell (1959), p. 64.
3. SIECUS (1970), p. 122.
4. Hunt (1974), p. 142.
5. Child Study Association of America (1974).

BIBLIOGRAPHY

ABARBANEL, A. Nutrition, Health and Sexuality. In *Encyclopedia of Sexual Behavior* (A. Ellis and A. Abarbanel, Eds.). New York: Hawthorne, 1961.

ACHILLES, P. S. *The Effectiveness of Certain Social Hygiene Literature.* New York: Amer. Soc. Hyg. Assoc., 1923.

BACH, G. and WYDEN, P. *The Intimate Enemy.* New York: William Morrow, 1968.

BEACH, F. A Review of Physiological and Psychological Studies of Sexual Behavior in Mammals. *Physiol. Rev.* 27:240–307, 1947.

BECKER, R. Quiz. *Med Aspects of Human Sexuality.* September 1973.

BELMONT, H. Sex Education of the Child and Adolescent. In *Sexual Function and Dysfunction.* (P. Fink and V. Hammett, Eds.). Philadelphia: F. A. Davis, 1969.

BERGLER, E. *Neurotic Counterfeit Sex.* New York: Grune and Stratton, 1951.

BERGLER, E. and KROGER, W. S. *Kinsey's Myth of Female Sexuality.* New York: Grune and Stratton, 1954.

BONAPARTE, M. *Female Sexuality.* New York: International Universities Press, 1953.

BONAPARTE, M. Passivity, Masochism and Femininity. *Int. J. Psychoanal.* 16:325–333, 1935.

BRECHER, E., *The Sex Researchers*. Boston: Little, Brown, 1969.

BROMLEY, D. D. and BRITTEN, F. H. *Youth and Sex. A Study of College Students*. New York: Harper, 1938.

BROWN, D. Female Orgasm and Sexual Inadequacy. In *An Analysis of Human Sexual Response* (E. Brecher, Ed.). New York: New American Library, 1966.

BRYK, F. *Circumcision in Man and Woman*. New York: Amer. Ethnological Press, 1934.

BURNS, R. K. Role of Hormones in the Differentiation of Sex. In *Sex and Internal Secretions* (W. C. Young, Ed.). Baltimore: Williams and Wilkins, 1961.

BYCHOWSKI, G. Some Aspects of Psychosexuality in Psychoanalytic Experience. In *Psychosexual Development in Health and Disease*. (P. H. Hoch and J. Zubin, Eds.) New York: Grune and Stratton, 1949.

CALDERONE, M. Conception Control and Sexual Problems. In *Sexual Problems: Diagnosis and Treatment in Medical Practice* (C. Wahl, Ed.). New York: Macmillan, 1967.

CAMERON, D. E. Sexuality and Sexual Disorders. In *Modern Practice in Psychological Medicine* (J. R. Rees, Ed.). New York: Hoeber, 1960.

CHESLER, P. *Women and Madness*. New York: Avon, 1972.

Child Study Association of America. Wel-Met Incorporated. *What to Tell Your Child About Sex*. New York: Pocket Books, 1974.

CLARK, L. Adhesions Between Clitoris and Prepuce. In *Advances in Sex Research* (H. Biegel, Ed.). New York: Hoeber, 1963.

*CLARK, L. *101 Intimate Sexual Problems Answered*. New York, New American Library, 1968.

CLARK, L. *101 More Intimate Sexual Problems Answered*. New York: New American Library, 1968.

CLARK, L. *The Enjoyment of Love in Marriage*. New York: New American Library, 1969.

COMFORT, A. (Trans.). *Koka Shastra*. New York: Ballantine Books, 1961.

COMFORT, A. (Ed.). *The Joy of Sex*. New York: Crown, 1972.

COMFORT, A. (Ed.). *More Joy*. New York: Crown, 1974.

Commission on Obscenity and Pornography. *Report of the*

Commission on Obscenity and Pornography. New York: Bantam, 1970.

CURTIS, A., ANSON, B. and McVAY, C. The Anatomy of the Pelvic and Urogenital Diaphragms in Relation to Urethrocoele and Cystocoele. *Surg, Gynec., Obstet.* 68:161–166, 1939.

DAVIS, K. B. *Factors in the Sex Life of Twenty-Two Hundred Women.* New York: Harper, 1929.

DEARBORN, L. W. Autoeroticism. In *Encyclopedia of Sexual Behavior* (A. Ellis and A. Abarbanel, Eds.). New York: Hawthorne, 1961.

DEBEAUVOIR, S. *The Second Sex.* New York: Knopf, 1952.

DEUTSCH, H. *The Psychology of Women.* Vols. I & II. New York: Grune and Stratton, 1945.

DEUTSCH, R. *The Key to Feminine Response in Marriage.* New York: Ballantine Books, 1968.

DICKINSON, R. L. *Atlas of Human Sex Anatomy.* Baltimore: Williams and Wilkins, 1949.

DICKINSON, R. L. and BEAM, L. *A Thousand Marriages.* Baltimore: Williams and Wilkins, 1931.

DICKINSON, R. L. and BEAM, L. *The Single Woman.* Baltimore: Williams and Wilkins, 1934.

DICKINSON, R. L. and PIERSON, H. H. The Average Sex Life of American Women. *J.A.M.A.* 85:1113–1117, 1925.

EISSLER, K. On Certain Problems of Female Sexual Development. *Psychoanal. Quart.* 8:191–210, 1939.

*ELLIS, A. *Sex Without Guilt.* New York: Lyle Stuart, 1966.

ELLIS, H. *Psychology of Sex: A Manual for Students.* New York: New Amer. Lib., 1933.

EXNER, M. J. *Problems and Principles of Sex Education.* New York: Association Press, 1915.

FENICHEL, O. *The Psychoanalytic Theory of Neurosis.* New York: Norton, 1945.

FINGER, F. W. Sex Beliefs and Practices Among Male College Students. *J. Abn. Soc. Psych.* 42:57–67.

FINK, P. A Review of the Investigations of Masters and Johnson. In *Sexual Function and Dysfunction* (P. Fink and V. Hammett, Eds.). Philadelphia: F. A. Davis, 1969.

FISHER, S. *The Female Orgasm: Psychology, Physiology, Fantasy.* New York: Basic Books, 1973.

FISHER, S. *Understanding the Female Orgasm*. New York: Bantam, 1973.

FORD, C. Culture and Sex. In *The Encyclopedia of Sexual Behavior* (A. Ellis and A. Abarbanel, Eds.). New York, Hawthorne, 1961.

FORD, C. and BEACH, F. *Patterns of Sexual Behavior*. New York: Harper and Row, 1951.

FREUD, S. Beyond the Pleasure Principle. In *Complete Psychological Works of Sigmund Freud* (Standard Ed.) (J. Strachey, Trans.). Vol. 18. London: Hogarth Press, 1955.

FREUD, S. *New Introductory Lectures on Psychoanalysis* (W. J. H. Sprott, Trans.). New York: W. W. Norton, 1933.

FREUD, S. Three Contributions to the Theory of Sex: The Transformation of Puberty. In *The Basic Writings of Sigmund Freud* (A.A. Brill, Trans. and Ed.). New York: Random House, 1938.

FREUD, S. *The Sexual Enlightenment of Children*. New York: Collier Books, 1963. (First published in 1907 in *Soziale Medizin and Hygiene*, Bd. II, 1907 as an "open letter" to the editor, Dr. M. Furst.)

GAGINON, J. and SIMON, W. Sex Education and Human Development. In *Sexual Function and Dysfunction* (P. Fink and V. Hammett, Eds.). Philadelphia: F. A. Davis, 1969.

GLADWIN, T. and SARASON, S. *Truk: Man in Paradise*. New York: Werner-Gren Foundation, 1953.

GOLDSTEIN, M., HAEBERLE, E. and McBRIDE, W. *The Sex Book*. New York: Herder and Herder, 1971.

GRABER, B. and KLINE-GRABER, G. Clitoral Foreskin Adhesions: Description, Incidence, and Technique for Surgical Lysis. Presented at National Meeting Soc. Scientific Study Sex, August, 1974.

GRABER, B. and KLINE-GRABER, G. Epidermiological Report on Clitoral Foreskin Adhesions. Presented at Second Annual Conference Sex Therapists and Counselors. Galveston, Texas, March 1975.

GREENBANK, R. K. Are Medical Students Learning Psychiatry? *Med. J.* 64:989–992, 1961.

GUTTMACHER, A. *Birth Control and Love*. New York: Bantam Books, 1970.

HAMILTON, E. Emotions and Sexuality in the Woman. In *The*

New Sexuality (H. Otto, Ed.). Palo Alto: Science and Behavior Books, 1971.

HAMPSON, J. and HAMPSON, J. Ontogenesis of Sexual Behavior in Man. In *Sex and Internal Secretions* (W. C. Young, Ed.). Baltimore: Williams and Wilkins, 1961.

HARDENBERGH, E. W. The Psychology of Feminine Sex Experience. In *Sex, Society and the Individual* (A. P. Pillay and A. Ellis, Eds.). Bombay, India: *Int. J. Sex.*, 1953.

HARLOW, H. Sexual Behavior in the Rhesus Monkey. In *Sex and Behavior* (F. Beach, Ed.). New York: Wiley and Sons, 1965.

*HASTINGS, D. W. *A Doctor Speaks on Sexual Expression in Marriage.* Boston: Little, Brown, 1966.

HASTINGS, D. W. Lack of Sex Sensation. In *Sexual Freedom in Marriage* (L. Rubin, Ed.). New York: New American Library, 1969.

HITSCHMANN, E. and BERGLER, E. Frigidity in Women: Restatement and Renewed Experience. *Psychoanal. Rev.* 36:45–53, 1949.

HORNEY, K. The Denial of the Vagina: A Contribution to the Problem of the Genital Anxieties Specific to Women. *Int. J. Psychoanal.* 14:55–70, 1933.

HUGHES, W. L. Sex Experiences of Boyhood. *J. Soc. Hyg.* 12:262–273, 1926.

HUNT, M. *Sexual Behavior in the Seventies.* Chicago: Playboy Press, 1974.

HUXLEY, A. *The Doors of Perception.* New York: Harper and Row, 1954.

JONG, E. *Fear of Flying.* New York: Holt, Rinehart and Winston, 1973.

KAGAN, J. Acquisition and Significance of Sex Typing and Sex Role Identity. In *Review of Child Development and Research* (M. L. Hoffman and L. Hoffman, Eds.). New York: Russel Sage Foundation, 1964.

KANE, F. Psychoendocrine Study of Oral Contraceptive Agents. *Am. J. of Psych.* 127:443–50, October 1970.

KAPLAN, H. K. *Sex Behavior*, September 1972.

KAPLAN, H. K. *The New Sex Therapy.* New York: Brunner/Mazel, 1974.

KEGEL, A. and POWELL, T. The Physiologic Treatment of Urinary Stress Incontinence. *J. of Urol.* 63:808–813, 1950.

KEGEL, A. The Non-Surgical Treatment of Genital Relaxation. *Ann of West Med. and Surg.* 2:213–216, 1948.

KEGEL, A. Progressive Resistance Exercise in the Functional Restoration of the Perineal Muscles. *Am. J. of Obst. and Gyn.* 56:238–248, 1948.

KEGEL, A. The Physiologic Treatment of Poor Tone and Function of the Genital Muscles and of Urinary Stress Incontinence. *West. J. of Surg., Obst. and Gyn.* 56:527–535, 1949.

KEGEL, A. Physiologic Therapy for Urinary Stress Incontinence. *J.A.M.A.* 146:915–917, 1951.

KEGEL, A. Stress Incontinence and Genital Relaxation. *CIBA Clin. Symposia* 4(2):35–51, February–March 1952.

KEGEL, A. Physiologic Therapy of Urinary Stress Incontinence. In *Monographs on Surgery 1952* (B. N. Carter, Ed.). Baltimore: Williams and Wilkins, 1952.

KEGEL, A. Sexual Functions of the Pubococcygeus Muscle. *West. J. of Surg., Obst, and Gyn.* 60:521–524, 1952.

KEGEL, A. Stress Incontinence of Urine in Women: Physiologic Treatment, *J. of Intl. Coll. Surg.* XXV:487–499, 1956.

KEGEL, A. Early Genital Relaxation. *Obst. and Gyn.* 8:545–550, 1956.

KINSEY, A. C. et al. *Sexual Behavior in the Human Male.* Philadelphia, W. B. Saunders, 1948.

KINSEY, A. C. et al. *Sexual Behavior in the Human Female.* Philadelphia: W. B. Saunders, 1953.

KIRKENDALL, L. Sex Drive. In *Encyclopedia of Sexual Behavior* (A. Ellis and A. Abarbanel, Eds.). New York: Hawthorne, 1961.

KLEEGMAN, J. Clinical Applications of Masters and Johnson's Research. In *Sexual Function and Dysfunction* (P. Fink and V. Hammett, Eds.). Philadelphia: F. A. Davis, 1969.

KLEMER, R. Female Sexual Conditioning. In *Counseling in Marital and Sexual Problems* (R. Klemer, Ed.). Baltimore: Williams and Wilkins, 1965.

KLINE-GRABER, G. and GRABER, B. The Use of Pubococcygeus Exercises to Improve Vaginal Sensation. Unpublished, 1974.

KLINE-GRABER, G. and GRABER, B. The Pubococcygeus Muscle and Sexual Functioning: An Update on Kegel's

Work. Presented at Second Annual Conference Sex Therapists and Counselors. Galveston, Texas, March 1975.

KNIGHT, R. P. Functional Disturbances in the Sexual Life of Women. *Bull. of the Menninger Clinic* 7:25–35, 1943.

KOHLBERG, L. A. A Cognitive–Developmental Analysis of Children's Sex-Role Concepts and Attitudes. In *The Development of Sex Differences* (E. Maccogy, Ed.). Palo Alto: Stanford University Press, 1964.

KRANTZ, K. E. Physiology of Female Orgasm. *Med. Aspects Human Sex.* 7:11, March 1973.

KRANTZ, K. E. Innervation of the Human Vulva and Vagina. *Ob. Gyn.* 12:4, 1958.

KRAFFT-EBING, R. *Psychopathia Sexualis* (H. Wedeck, Trans.). New York: G. P. Putnam's Sons, 1965. (First published 1886.)

KROGER, W. S. and FREED, S. C. Psychosomatic Aspects of Frigidity. *J.A.M.A.* 143:526–532, 1950.

KRONHAUSEN, E. and KRONHAUSEN, P. *The Sexually Responsive Woman.* New York: Ballantine Books, 1964.

LAING, R. D. *The Politics of Experience.* New York: Ballantine Books, 1967.

LANDIS, J. T., POFFENBERGER, S. and POFFENBERGER, J. The Effects of First Pregnancy Upon the Sexual Adjustment of 212 Couples. *Amer. Soc. Review.* 15:676–772, 1950.

LAZARUS, A. *Behavior Therapy and Beyond.* New York: McGraw-Hill, 1971.

LIEF, H. Sex Education of the Physician. In *Sexual Function and Dysfunction* (P. Fink and V. Hammett, Eds.). Philadelphia: F. A. Davis, 1969.

LLEWELLYN-JONES, D. *Everywoman and Her Body.* New York: Lancer, 1971.

LoPICCOLO, J. and LOBITZ, M. A. The Role of Masturbation in the Treatment of Orgasmic Dysfunction. *Arch. of Sex. Behavior.* 2:163–171, 1972.

LoPICCOLO, J. and LOBITZ, W. G. Behavior Therapy of Sexual Dysfunction. Presented at Fourth Intl. Conf. on Behavior. Banff, Alberta, Canada, 1972.

LOWEN, A. Movement and Feeling in Sex. In *The Encyclopedia of Sexual Behavior* (A. Ellis and A. Abarbanel, Eds.). New York: Hawthorne, 1961.

LOWEN, A. *Pleasure.* New York: Lancer, 1970.

LUNDBERG, F. and FARNHAM, M. *Modern Woman, the Lost Sex.* New York: Harper, 1967.

MARSHALL, D. Sexual Behavior on Mangaia. In *Human Sexual Behavior* (D. Marshall and R. Suggs, Eds.). Englewood Cliffs: Prentice-Hall, 1971.

MASTERS, W. H. The Sex Response Cycle of the Human Female. *West. J. Surg., Obst. and Gyn.* 68:57–72, 1960.

MASTERS, W. H. The Sex Response Cycle of the Human Female: II. Vaginal Lubrication. *Ann. N. Y. Acad. Sci.* 83:301–317, 1959.

MASTERS, W. H. and JOHNSON, V. E. The Human Female: Anatomy of Sexual Response, *Minn. Med.* 43:31–36, January 1960.

MASTERS, W. H. and JOHNSON, V. E. Orgasm, Anatomy of the Female. In *The Encyclopedia of Sexual Behavior* (A. Ellis and A. Abarbanel, Eds.). New York: Hawthorne Books, 1961.

MASTERS, W. H. and JOHNSON, V. E. The Sexual Response Cycle of the Human Female: III. The Clitoris: Anatomic and Clinical Considerations. *West. J. Surg., Obst. and Gyn.* 70:248–257, 1962.

MASTERS, W. H. and JOHNSON, V. E. Counseling with Sexually Incompatible Marriage Partners. In *Counseling in Marital and Sexual Problems* (R. H. Klemer, Ed.). Baltimore: Williams and Wilkins, 1965.

MASTERS, W. H. and JOHNSON, V. E. *Human Sexual Response.* Boston: Little, Brown, 1966.

MASTERS, W. H. and JOHNSON, V. E. *Human Sexual Inadequacy.* Boston: Little, Brown, 1970.

MAXWELL, R. J. Quiz: Female Sexuality in Primitive Cultures. *Med. Aspects Human Sex.* 1:193, January 1973.

McGOVERN, K., STEWART, R. and LoPICCOLO, J. Secondary Orgasmic Dysfunction I: Analysis and Strategies for Treatment (unpublished).

McGUIRE, T. and STEINHILBER, R. Sexual Frigidity. *Mayo Clin. Proc.* 39:416–426, 1964.

MEAD, M. *Male ad Female.* New York: William Morrow, 1949.

MEAD, M. Cultural Determinants of Sexual Behavior. In *Sex and Internal Secretions* (W. C. Young, Ed.). Baltimore: Williams and Wilkins, 1961.

MEADE, M. If She's Passive, You May Be Missing Something. *Sexology.* October 1973.

MIKUTA, J. and PAYNE, F. Stress Urinary Incontinence in the Female. A Review of the Modern Approach to This Problem. *Amer. J. Med. Sci.* 226:674–686, 1953.

MONEY, J. *Man and Woman, Boy and Girl.* Baltimore: Johns Hopkins University Press, 1972.

NEIGER, S. Does Sex Know-How Come Naturally? *Sexology.* October 1973.

NEIGER, S. The Importance of Good Sex Hygiene. In *Sexual Expression in Marriage* (I. Rubin, Ed.). New York: New America Library, 1969.

OLIVEN, J. *Sexual Hygiene and Pathology.* Philadelphia: Lippincott, 1965.

O'NEILL, G. and O'NEILL, N. *Open Marriage.* New York: M. Evans, 1972.

OTTO, H. and OTTO, R. *Total Sex.* New York: Wyden, 1972.

PEARL, R. *The Biology of Population Growth.* New York: Alfred A. Knopf, 1925.

PECK, M. W. and WELLS, F. L. On the Psycho-Sexuality of College Graduate Men. *Ment. Hyg.* 7:697–714, October 1923.

PECK, M. W. and WELLS, F. L. Further Studies in the Psycho-Sexuality of College Graduate Men. *Ment. Hyg.* 9:502–520, July 1925.

POMEROY, W. *Girls and Sex.* New York: Delacorte Press, 1969.

POMEROY, W. *Dr. Kinsey and the Institute for Sex Research.* New York: The New American Library, 1972.

POTTS, M. and PEEL, J. *Textbook of Contraceptive Practice.* Cambridge, Great Britain; Cambridge University Press, 1970.

RADO, S. Sexual Anaesthesia in the Female. *Quart. Rev. Surg. Obst. and Gyn.* 16:249–253, 1959.

RAINWATER, L. *Family Design. Marital Sexuality, Family Size, and Contraception.* Chicago: Aldine Publishers, 1965.

RATHMANN, W. G. Female Circumcision, Indications and a New Technique. *General Practice.* XX:115–120, 1959.

REICH, W. *The Function of the Orgasm.* New York: World Publishing, 1971.

REICH, W. *The Sexual Revolution.* New York. Farrar, Straus, and Giroux, 1969.

ROBINSON, M. *The Power of Sexual Surrender.* Garden City: Doubleday, 1959.

RUSSELL, B. *Marriage. and Morals.* New York: Bantam, 1959. (Orig. Pub. New York: H. Liveright, 1929).

SEAMAN, B. *Free and Female.* Greenwich: Fawcett, 1972.

SEMMENS, J. Questions and Answers. *Med. Aspects Human Sex.* 7:10, 11, 159–169, March 1973.

Sex Information and Education Council of the United States. *Sexuality and Man.* New York: Scribner's, 1970.

SHERFEY, M. J. The Evolution and Nature of Female Sexuality in Relation to Psychoanalytic Theory. *J. Amer. Psychoanal. Assoc.* 14(1):28–128, 1966.

SHERFEY, M. J. *The Nature and Evolution of Female Sexuality.* New York: Random House, 1966.

STEKEL, W. *Frigidity in Woman in Relation to Her Love Life.* Vols. I and II. New York: Liveright, 1926.

STEKEL, W. *Auto Eroticism: A Psychiatric Study of Orgasm and Neurosis.* New York: Liveright, 1950.

STONE, A. and STONE, H. *A Marriage Manual,* New York: Simon and Schuster, 1952. (Rev. ed. Orig. ed. 1935.)

STOKES, W. Control of Procreation: A New Dimension of Freedom. In *The New Sexuality* (H. Otto, Ed.). Palo Alto: Science and Behavior Books, 1971.

TERMAN, L. M. *Psychological Factors in Marital Happiness.* New York: McGraw Hill, 1938.

THOMPSON, C. *On Women* (M. Green, Ed.). New York: Basic Books, 1964.

TISSOT, S. A. *L'Onanisme: Dissertation sur les Maladies Produites par la Masturbation.* Lausanne: Marc Chapiuse et Cie. XXIV, 1764.

VAN DE VELDE, T. H. *Ideal Marriage.* New York: Random House, 1930.

WALLIN, P. and CLARK, A. A Study of Orgasm as a Condition of Women's Enjoyment of Coitus in the Middle Years of Marriage. *Human. Biol.* 35:131–139, 1963.

WEISS, E. and ENGLISH, O. S. *Psychosomatic Medicine.* Philadelphia: Saunders, 1949.

WHARTON, L. The Non-Operative Treatment of Stress Incontinence in Women. *J. of Urol.* 69(4):511–519, 1953.

WILBUR, D. Scientific Revolution Is Near. *Amer. Med. Assoc. News.* Pg. 1, May 5, 1969.

WOLFE, L. Take Two Aspirins and Masturbate. *Playboy* 21:6, September 1974.

WOLPE, J. *The Practice of Behavior Therapy.* New York: Pergamon, 1969.

WRIGHT, H. A Contribution to the Orgasm Problem in Women. In *Sex, Society and the Individual* (A. P. Pillay and A. Ellis, Eds.). Bombay, India: *Int. J. Sex.,* 1953.

YOUNG, W. C. The Hormones and Mating Behavior. In *Sex and Internal Secretions* (W. C. Young, Ed.). Baltimore: Williams and Wilkins, 1961.

Index